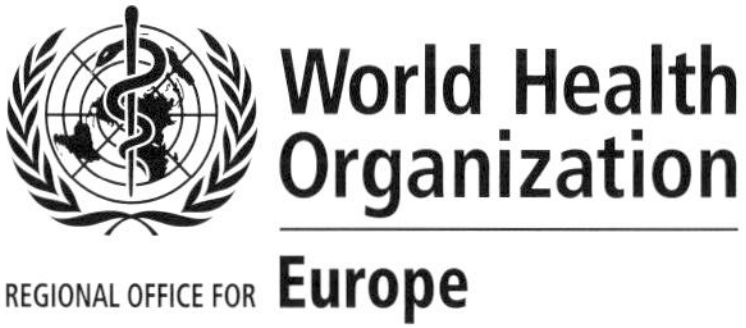

# European report on preventing elder maltreatment

Edited by *Dinesh Sethi, Sara Wood, Francesco Mitis, Mark Bellis, Bridget Penhale, Isabel Iborra Marmolejo, Ariela Lowenstein, Gillian Manthorpe & Freja Ulvestad Kärki*

# Abstract

Elder maltreatment is pervasive in all countries in the WHO European Region, and estimates suggest that at least 4 million people in the Region experience elder maltreatment in any one year. Most countries in the Region have an ageing population, and one third of the population is forecast to be 60 years and older in 2050, putting more people at risk of elder maltreatment. Elder maltreatment has far-reaching consequences for the mental and physical well-being of tens of millions of older people, and if left unchecked will result in their premature death. Estimates suggest that about 2500 older people may lose their lives annually from elder maltreatment. The report highlights the numerous biological, social, cultural, economic and environmental factors that interact to influence the risk and protective factors of being a victim or perpetrator of elder maltreatment. There is some evidence of effectiveness, and examples include psychological programmes for perpetrators and programmes designed to change attitudes towards older people, improve the mental health of caregivers and, in earlier life, to promote nurturing relationships and social skills learning. The evidence base needs to be strengthened, but much can be done by implementing interventions using an evaluative framework. Prevention and social justice for older people can only be achieved by mainstreaming this response into health and social policy. Surveys show that the public and policy-makers are increasingly concerned about the problem, and the policy response needs to be strengthened to meet this demand.

Keywords
ELDER ABUSE - prevention and control
AGGRESSION
INTERGENERATIONAL RELATIONS
AGED
EUROPE

ISBN 978 92 890 0237 0

Address requests about publications of the WHO Regional Office for Europe to:
Publications
WHO Regional Office for Europe
Scherfigsvej 8
DK-2100 Copenhagen Ø, Denmark

Alternatively, complete an online request form for documentation, health information, or for permission to quote or translate, on the Regional Office web site (http://www.euro.who.int/pubrequest).



Text editing: David Breuer
Design: Møller & Kompagni
Printed in Rome, Italy by Servizi Tipografici Carlo Colombo

FRONT COVER PHOTO CREDIT
Istockphoto

INNER PHOTO CREDITS
Istockphoto: pp. 2, 3, 4, 25, 29, 31, 32, 33, 36, 37, 43, 46, 47, 50, 52, 60, 66
WHO/Matthias Braubach: p. 9
WHO/Chris Black: p. 64
Centro Reina Sofia/Ivana Maritano: p. 23
Centro Reina Sofia/Miren Eguzkiñe Egaña Corta: p. 35 (left)
Centro Reina Sofia/Santiago Burgos Mateo: p. 35 (right)
Centro Reina Sofia/Víctor Seguí Pruñonosa: p. 51

# Contents

# Acronyms

| | |
|---|---|
| ABUEL | Abuse and health among elderly in Europe |
| CIS | Commonwealth of Independent States |
| DALYs | Disability-adjusted life-years |
| EU | European Union |
| HALE | Healthy life expectancy |

# Acknowledgements

Many international experts and WHO staff members have contributed to developing this publication, and we are very thankful for their support and guidance. The conceptual foundations for this publication were outlined at a meeting held in London during the SAFETY 2010 Conference. Consultation participants included Alexander Butchart, Nancy M. Gage-Lindner, Christiane Hauzeur, Dimitrinka Jordanova-Pesevska, Freja Ulvestad Kärki, Fanka Koycheva, Francesco Mitis, Bridget Penhale, Marija Raleva, Dinesh Sethi, Marie Svendsen and Fimka Tozija. Ideas were further developed at an editorial meeting held in Rome on 14–15 February 2011 when the following were present: Thomas Goergen, Dimitrinka Jordanova-Pesevska, Freja Ulvestad Kärki, Ariela Lowenstein, Gillian Manthorpe, Christopher Mikton, Francesco Mitis, Bridget Penhale, Francesca Racioppi, Marija Raleva, Dinesh Sethi and Sara Wood.

We are particularly grateful to the following WHO staff members:

- Enrique Loyola and Ivo Rakovac for providing advice and data from WHO mortality and hospital admissions databases;
- Alexander Butchart for providing very useful comments and sharing references;
- Colin Mathers for providing information on healthy life expectancy;
- Manfred Huber for providing very helpful comments;
- Dany Berluteau Tsouros and Patricia Søndergaard for help in obtaining references;
- Nicoletta Di Tanno for help in searching for and selecting photographs;
- Manuela Gallitto for administrative support;
- Srdan Matic for support and encouragement; and
- Francesca Racioppi for support, encouragement and thorough and helpful comments on initial drafts.

We are particularly grateful to our external peer reviewers for their very helpful comments and for contributing to improving the completeness and accuracy of this publication:

- Maria Teresa Bazo, Universidad del País Vasco, Bilbao, Spain;
- Jeffrey E. Hall and Debra Karch, Centers for Disease Control and Prevention, Atlanta, United States of America; and
- Gloria M. Gutman, Simon Fraser University Gerontology Research Centre, Vancouver, Canada.

We thank:

- Robert Bauer, Austrian Road Safety Board, Vienna, Austria for providing data from the EU Injury Database;
- Joaquim J.F. Soares, Karolinska Institutet, and Maria Gabriella Melchiorre, Italian National Institute of Health and Science on Aging, Ancona, for material and information on the Abuse and health among elderly in Europe (ABUEL) project;
- Gabiele Meyer, University of Witten/Herdecke for information on intervention studies; and
- Gianfranco Salvioli, University of Modena, for information and material on elder maltreatment and care workers in Italy.

We are very grateful to the health ministry focal people for violence prevention who participated in the survey on the prevention of elder maltreatment and to the heads of country offices who helped coordinate the national responses.

Finally we thank Gauden Galea, Director, Division of Noncommunicable Diseases and Guenael Rodier, Director, Division of Communicable Diseases, Health Security and Environment, WHO Regional Office for Europe, for encouragement and support.

Dinesh Sethi was the lead editor. Sara Wood, Francesco Mitis, Mark Bellis, Bridget Penhale, Isabel Iborra Marmolejo, Ariela Lowenstein, Gillian Manthorpe and Freja Ulvestad Kärki contributed to the editing. The authorship of the chapters is as follows:

- Chapter 1: Dinesh Sethi and Francesco Mitis
- Chapter 2: Dinesh Sethi, Francesco Mitis, Thomas Görgen and Freja Ulvestad Kärki
- Chapter 3: Isabel Iborra Marmolejo and Bridget Penhale
- Chapter 4: Sara Wood, Mark Bellis and Christopher Mikton

- Chapter 5: Ariela Lowenstein, Gillian Manthorpe, Dinesh Sethi and Francesco Mitis
- Annexes: Francesco Mitis and Dinesh Sethi

We are grateful to the following experts for contributing valuable case studies of elder maltreatment in the WHO European Region:

- Box 1.2: Thomas Görgen
- Box 5.2: Dimitrinka Jordanova-Pesevska and Marija Raleva.

Thomas Görgen also shared valuable information and insights on programmes and policy.

The WHO Regional Office for Europe thanks the Department of Health in England and the Government of the United Kingdom for their generous support.

*Dinesh Sethi, Sara Wood, Francesco Mitis, Mark Bellis, Bridget Penhale, Isabel Iborra Marmolejo, Ariela Lowenstein, Gillian Manthorpe and Freja Ulvestad Kärki*

# Foreword

*Elder maltreatment is pervasive in all countries in the European Region. It is a growing concern, and estimates suggest that at least 4 million people experience elder maltreatment in any one year in the Region. The full scale of the problem is not properly understood, but it has far-reaching consequences for the mental and physical well-being of tens of millions of older people and, if left unchecked, may result in their premature death. Most countries in the Region have an ageing population, and one third of the population is forecast to be 60 years and older in 2050, putting more people at risk of elder maltreatment. Much of old age is a healthy period, although there may be disability and dependence requiring family and societal support, especially in late old age. The current economic downturn has put more strain on these support structures in the Region, which in turn may put more older people at risk of maltreatment. Elder maltreatment is a health and social problem, and preventing it is an issue of human rights and social solidarity.*

*This has resulted in increasing concern among the public and policy-makers about elder maltreatment. Scientific evidence from Europe and elsewhere is increasing on the scale, causes and grave effects of the problem and what can be done to prevent it. Nevertheless, more resources need to be devoted to developing and implementing strategies to reduce elder maltreatment. There is some initial promising evidence in some areas, such as training and supporting professional and family caregivers and promoting positive attitudes towards older people. Reducing the cycles of violence by investing in nurturing relationships and improving social cohesion across the generations is a worthwhile investment. Although the research evidence needs to be improved, numerous interventions could nevertheless be implemented through an evaluative framework. Ensuring that there is greater implementation through evaluative frameworks is one challenge facing policy-makers and practitioners, and responding to this requires concerted action.*

*The problem of elder maltreatment is a common challenge across government departments and a shared problem that cuts across the activity areas of many sectors. Health systems have a key role to play in providing services for victims of maltreatment who have been harmed physically and mentally. The health sector is also best placed to advocate for preventive approaches with an evaluative framework. Decisive action is needed now to fill these gaps in research and to take effective steps to secure the safety and well-being of older people in the European Region. Prevention and social justice for older people can only be achieved by mainstreaming the response into other areas of health and social policy.*

*We invite Member States of the European Region to join the global effort to reduce a leading health and social problem and to create safer and more just societies for older people. We at WHO hope that this report will provide policy-makers, practitioners and activists with the facts needed to integrate the agenda for preventing elder maltreatment both within and outside the health sector.*

Zsuzsanna Jakab

WHO Regional Director for Europe

# Executive summary

Elder maltreatment is physical, sexual, mental and/or financial abuse and/or neglect of people aged 60 years and older. The scale of the problem of elder maltreatment has not been properly defined, but estimates indicate that at least 4 million older people experience it in any one year in the WHO European Region. With the ageing population in the Region, the numbers affected by elder maltreatment are likely to increase, and this highlights the need for action to be taken to halt this potential increase. Elder maltreatment affects both the mental and physical well-being of older people and, if unchecked, leads to poorer quality of life and reduced survival. It is thus an important public health problem. Further, preventing elder maltreatment is an issue of human rights and social solidarity. Society has an obligation to preserve the rights of older people, which may be eroded by ageism in the form of negative societal attitudes towards older people and stereotypes. To overcome this, social cohesion and solidarity across generations needs to be strengthened. Prevention programmes need to be put in place and a public health approach informed by evidence is needed to meet this challenge.

### Population at risk

Life expectancy is increasing in most countries in the Region and the populations are therefore ageing rapidly. In 2050, one third of the population is projected to be 60 years and older. This ageing population will put more older people at risk of maltreatment. Whereas much of old age is a healthy period, there may be ill health, which leads to disability and dependence, especially in late old age. This may increase the demands on family caregivers and the need for a trained health and social care workforce. This is particularly the case in supporting people with dementia and multiple problems. Many older people have reduced incomes, which increases their dependence on family and societal support. Older women have a much higher risk of poverty than older men. The current economic downturn has put more strain on these support structures in Europe, and older people living in deprived neighbourhoods are likely to be more at risk.

### Why is preventing elder maltreatment a priority in the European Region?

Older people are at risk from interpersonal violence, and 8500 people aged 60 years and older die from homicide annually in the WHO European Region. Interpersonal violence is an important cause of great inequality in health, and 9 of 10 homicide deaths among older people are in low- and middle-income countries. Assaults affecting older people are more common in sections of society that are more socioeconomically deprived. Elder maltreatment leads to an estimated 2500 (30%) annual homicides among older people; these are committed by family members. Information on fatal and nonfatal cases is grossly incomplete from routine databases in the Region, whether these are from the health, justice or social care sectors. The scale of the problem has only come to light by using population surveys in the community in the last few decades. Surveillance using routine information sources needs to be improved using standardized practices and definitions across all sectors and all countries.

The prevalence of elder maltreatment in the previous year in the community and other settings is high in the Region. Surveys of older people living in the community suggest that, in the previous year, about 2.7% of older people have experienced maltreatment in the form of physical abuse – equivalent to 4 million people aged 60 years and older in the Region. For sexual abuse, the proportion is lower at 0.7%, equivalent to 1 million older people; for mental abuse, this is far higher at 19.4%, equivalent to 29 million older people; and 3.8% have been subjected to financial abuse, equivalent to 6 million older people. It is therefore important to define the type of maltreatment being measured. The prevalence of elder maltreatment increases among people with disability, cognitive impairment and dependence, and reports suggest that this may be much higher among older disabled people with high support needs. The prevalence of elder maltreatment varies according to culture and country, and using more standardized definitions, instruments and methods would make European surveys more comparable. Surveys of family caregivers and professional caregivers show that large proportions report having maltreated older people in their care. These approaches could be better exploited to understand the scale of the problem of elder maltreatment. Elder maltreatment may lead to lasting harmful physical and mental effects among older people. The societal costs of elder maltreatment are thought to be high but need to be better studied in the Region.

### What are the risk and protective factors for elder maltreatment?

Numerous biological, social, cultural, economic and environmental factors interact to influence the risk of being a victim or perpetrator of elder maltreatment. Studies show that older people with dementia and with a disability that results in increased dependence on caregivers increases the risk of elder maltreatment. Similarly, living in the same household as the perpetrator also increases the risk. Perpetration is most often carried out by caregivers who are partners, offspring or other relatives, although professional health and care workers and visitors can also be perpetrators in institutions or at home. Perpetrators are more likely to have mental health problems, especially depression or a history of violence, and may suffer from substance misuse, especially alcohol abuse.

The latter may increase the perpetrator's financial dependence on older people. Increased dependence of the perpetrator on the victim, either financially or emotionally, increases the risk. One of the factors that appears to be important is the past quality of the relationship between the perpetrator and victim before the onset of maltreatment. Further, social isolation and not being part of social networks will also put older people at greater risk. Income and social inequality are risk factors for violence, and some evidence indicates that this is also the case for elder maltreatment. Social and cultural norms such as ageism, tolerance of violence and gender inequality may reinforce maltreatment in society and need to be better studied. The characteristics of institutions in which elder maltreatment has occurred have been described and include poor training and support of staff, tolerance of violence in the institution, inadequate support for activities of daily living and a lack of respect for and lack of autonomy among residents.

Protective factors such as positive life experiences and community connectedness seem to prevent and mitigate the effects of maltreatment and should be promoted. Having visitors and relatives visiting residents appears to protect older people in care homes from maltreatment.

Further, the role of perpetrators' previous exposure to violence in perpetuating the cycles of violence needs to be better understood, and the intergenerational effects of earlier exposure to interpersonal violence on perpetration needs to be examined. High-quality research studies of risk and protective factors pertaining to elder maltreatment are lacking, both within the European Region and elsewhere. These would assist in developing and targeting strategies to prevent and intervene in situations of elder maltreatment.

## What can be done to prevent elder maltreatment?

Numerous interventions have been implemented across Europe and globally to prevent and protect older people and to improve risk factors related to elder maltreatment. Although the evidence on which they are based is very often lacking, they nevertheless indicate that governments and nongovernmental organizations are giving this health and social problem greater priority and are beginning to address it. The lack of high-quality evaluation studies of interventions specifically designed to reduce or prevent elder maltreatment substantially limits conclusions about which interventions may be most effective.

The review of the evidence shows mixed findings for the effectiveness in reducing elder maltreatment of: professional awareness and education courses; legal, psychological and educational support programmes; and restraint reduction programmes. More research is needed to clarify the positive effects of these interventions. Evidence is emerging of effectiveness for psychological programmes for perpetrators, which have been associated with a reduction in self-reported abusive behaviour. However, further high-quality evaluations of these programmes are needed to provide a better understanding of potential effects. Further, promising evidence supports the use of programmes designed to change attitudes towards older people or improve caregiver mental health, but the effects on reduced elder maltreatment as an outcome have not yet been measured. Some interventions have been studied to show that they are associated with an apparent increase in reported maltreatment, and whether this results from better reporting or possibly even worse outcomes needs to be further clarified. The weak evidence base of what works needs to be improved. Further research is also needed on the costs associated with implementing elder maltreatment interventions. Policy-makers and practitioners should ensure that whenever possible, programmes should be implemented using an evaluative framework that includes elder maltreatment outcomes, longer term follow-up and measures of cost–effectiveness. More general strategies for preventing violence, such as those designed to create safe, nurturing parent–child relationships and equipping children and young people with the social skills necessary to successfully navigate through life are also likely to be important in preventing elder maltreatment, and long-term studies are needed to delineate whether this is the case.

## The way forward in the European Region

This report highlights the great public health and social problem that elder maltreatment presents, a problem that is likely to increase given the ageing population in the European Region. Literature is growing on the risk factors for elder maltreatment, and the evidence base of prevention programmes needs to be greatly improved, especially compared with other areas of interpersonal violence. Surveys show that the public and policy-makers are increasingly concerned about the problem. However, the policy response has been poor, and too few countries have devoted adequate resources to this growing public health priority. To improve on this inadequate response, this report proposes a set of actions for Member States, international agencies, nongovernmental organizations, researchers, practitioners and other stakeholders. These are in accordance with European Region and other international policy initiatives.

1. **Develop and implement national policies and plans for preventing elder maltreatment**

Health ministries need to take a leadership role in ensuring that national policies and plans for preventing elder maltreatment are developed. These should involve other ministries such as justice, education, social welfare, labour, environment and local planning. Efforts should be multidisciplinary, with broad representation from other sectors of government, and should involve nongovernmental organizations and older people.

2. **Take action to improve data on and surveillance of elder maltreatment**

All levels of data collection need to be improved, and agencies and countries need to share a common definition to better build national and local pictures of the scale of the problem. Such information is essential for developing evaluative frameworks for programme implementation and for advocacy.

3. **Evaluative research needs to be undertaken as a priority**

There is little rigorous knowledge of what works and for whom in preventing elder maltreatment and managing to minimize its harm. Systemic responses to primary prevention need to be developed as a priority, but good outcome research is needed to inform such decision-making. Researchers, donors and policy-makers need to intensify their efforts and make resources available to move the field ahead.

4. **Responses for victims need to be strengthened**

High-quality services need to be provided for victims of maltreatment for both physical and mental health outcomes. Health systems need to be strengthened to provide high-quality primary care services for the detection, management and referral of cases. A holistic approach to adult protective services with a clear evaluative framework is needed.

5. **Build capacity and exchange good practices across the sectors**

An essential part of an adequate service response is to ensure a supply of trained and experienced personnel who are well versed in detection, care and rehabilitation. This could be achieved by mainstreaming the prevention of elder maltreatment into the curricula of health professionals and other professionals from the justice, education and social care sectors. Older people need to be actively engaged in developing curricula.

6. **Address inequity in the maltreatment of older people**

The economic downturn in the European Region, the longer life expectancy and ageing population, the strain on social support services and increasing economic pressure on families and on older people themselves are exacerbating their vulnerability to elder maltreatment. Equity needs to be incorporated into all levels of government policy to address this cause of social injustice.

7. **Raise awareness and target investment for preventing elder maltreatment**

Raising awareness that maltreatment among older people should be prevented is paramount. The initial focus has been on protecting older people's dignity and their right not to be maltreated. Advocacy to prevent older people from being maltreated is needed throughout the European Region. Social marketing, mass media and education programmes should be used to raise awareness of the effects of maltreatment and to promote a healthy ageing approach to overcome negative stereotyping. Engaging older people in these processes is important.

8. **Protective factors, a life-course approach and intergenerational cohesion**

The demographic revolution in the European Region is accompanied by profound changes and presents fundamental challenges to social integration, social protection and social policies. A generational contract and innovative policy responses are therefore needed at the individual, familial, community and societal levels, with special emphasis on prevention. Relating to the different stages along the life course and how they affect family and care relations should be advocated.

9. **Ethics and the quality of services in the community and in institutions**

The health and social sectors are concerned with providing care for older people and with overseeing ethical standards and the quality of care for older people. Charters of rights are needed that provide standards that are binding for the organization and delivery of high-quality care.

# 1. Why elder maltreatment needs to be tackled in Europe

## 1.1 General introduction

There is increasing concern globally about the maltreatment of older people *(1)*. Elder maltreatment was regarded as a private matter until recently, and only in the last few decades have public health and criminal justice responses been developed to counter elder maltreatment *(2)*. The maltreatment of older people was first described in a letter in the British scientific press as "granny bashing" *(3,4)*. Since then, the health, social and justice sectors have shown increasing interest. Disquiet has been growing about the scale of the problem and the relative inaction worldwide and in the WHO European Region. This has been fuelled by the realization that the proportion of people aged 65 years and older globally is growing rapidly and that elder maltreatment will grow as a public health and societal problem. Further, there is concern that the economic downturn might exacerbate the risks as pressure increases on societal and family resources. Despite this, elder maltreatment is still a social taboo, and much of it is underreported and ignored in many countries in the WHO European Region.

The purpose of this report is:

- to describe the demographic changes occurring and discuss the scale of the problem of elder maltreatment in the WHO European Region;
- to identify risk factors and to examine the role of the social determinants of health;
- to describe the latest evidence on the effectiveness of interventions to prevent elder maltreatment;
- to identify experience in implementing evidence-informed programmes for preventing elder maltreatment in the European Region and elsewhere; and
- to identify strategies and key policy actions to reduce the burden of elder maltreatment, including for health systems in a multisectoral response.

## 1.2 What is elder maltreatment?

This report focuses on the maltreatment of people aged 60 years and older. Elder maltreatment is defined as a single or repeated act or lack of appropriate action, occurring within any relationship in which there is an expectation of trust, that causes harm or distress to older people *(1,5,6)*. Similar to other forms of violence,[1] elder maltreatment can take various forms of abuse such as physical, mental, emotional and sexual. It can also involve economic or financial abuse, in which other people inappropriately use older peoples' financial or related resources. Elder treatment can also be manifested as neglect.[2] Older people can be maltreated in the home, such as by family members, spouses, friends, caregivers or home care workers; or professionals or visitors can perpetrate elder maltreatment in institutional settings such as in nursing and residential homes and hospitals. Elder maltreatment would therefore by definition also include intimate partner violence, whether this is physical, sexual, mental or financial, among people aged 60 years and older. Elder maltreatment can also involve the use of physical restraints and overmedication to control behaviour, and professional care staff may carry this out in institutional settings, but caregivers or professional care staff may maltreat older people in their homes.

### Key facts

The European Region has a rapidly ageing population.

One third of the population of the European Region will be 60 years and older in 2050.

Many more older women than older men are in poverty.

The prevalence of elder maltreatment in the community is high (about 3%) and may be as high as 25% for older people with high support needs.

Societies define old age differently, and most countries in the European Region define old age to coincide with retirement at 60 or 65 years. In some countries, the retirement age is increasing. Studies may use different age categories and disaggregate data sets differently, but this report focuses on people aged 60 years and older wherever possible.

[1] The *World report on violence and health (1)* defines violence as the intentional use of physical force or power, threatened or actual, against oneself, another person, or against a group or community, that results either in injury, death, psychological harm, maldevelopment or deprivation. Violence may be classified as interpersonal when it occurs between individuals, as self-directed when directed to the self, or as collective violence which occurs between groups and may be politically or economically motivated. Many of the risk factors, however, are cross cutting and there are synergies in the strategies for prevention, whether they address interpersonal, self-directed or collective violence.

[2] Whereas most cases of maltreatment are intentional, intent may be difficult to determine. There is debate as to whether the definition of maltreatment should focus on adverse health and social outcomes instead of intent. Intention may be determined in many cases of maltreatment, though this can sometimes be difficult to distinguish, especially in cases of neglect.

## 1.3 Why is elder maltreatment a public health issue?

Elder maltreatment is a pervasive problem that affects all societies and countries. Little systematic study has been devoted to it, and routine information on the problem is scarce. Information from surveys in several countries suggests that 2.7% of older people in the general population report physical maltreatment in the previous month *(7)*. Intimate partner violence is reported by 5.6% of older people in the previous year *(8)*. For vulnerable adults requiring care, this is much higher, at 25%, and about one third of family caregivers report being involved in maltreatment. For nursing and residential homes for older people, the prevalence of maltreatment is much higher. Regardless of the setting, these high prevalence rates are of tremendous concern because maltreatment is associated with much pain and suffering and reduces the quality of life and shortens survival. Unfortunately, few routine data are available on the problem because of gross underrecording by health, police and social services *(9,10)*. This is partly because of underreporting of episodes of maltreatment by older people and/or caregivers and staff who might witness the situation. Older people who have been maltreated have longer hospital stays than those who have not been maltreated *(11,12)*.

Mortality data for homicide are usually complete in countries in the WHO European Region but may underrepresent the scale of the problem of elder maltreatment. The Global Burden of Disease study *(13)* reports 8300 people aged 60 years and older dying from homicide annually in the Region. As data on the relationship of the perpetrator to the victim are not routinely available, the numbers of homicides attributable to elder maltreatment cannot be accurately determined and need to be estimated. Research from several countries suggests that family members commit about 30% of homicides in this age group, which would therefore constitute elder maltreatment *(14,15)*. This suggests that about 2500 homicides annually can be attributed to elder maltreatment (see Annex 1 for methods). This may well be an underestimate, since insidious forms of maltreatment may go undetected.

Older people suffer violent deaths either directly – through homicide – or indirectly, through suicide, and premature mortality from other causes *(16)*. The overall disease burden is very high. In addition to the human costs, emerging evidence also shows that elder maltreatment has great economic costs, including the direct costs to health, social, legal, police and other services. Further, elder maltreatment also undermines efforts to improve older people's access to services and to social networks, thereby leaving them vulnerable to increased social isolation and ill health. Few European studies have been done, and one of the challenges for public health is to improve the evidence base on the causes and effects and the action needed to prevent maltreatment *(1)*. Further, the health sector and the social care sector are involved in providing care for older people

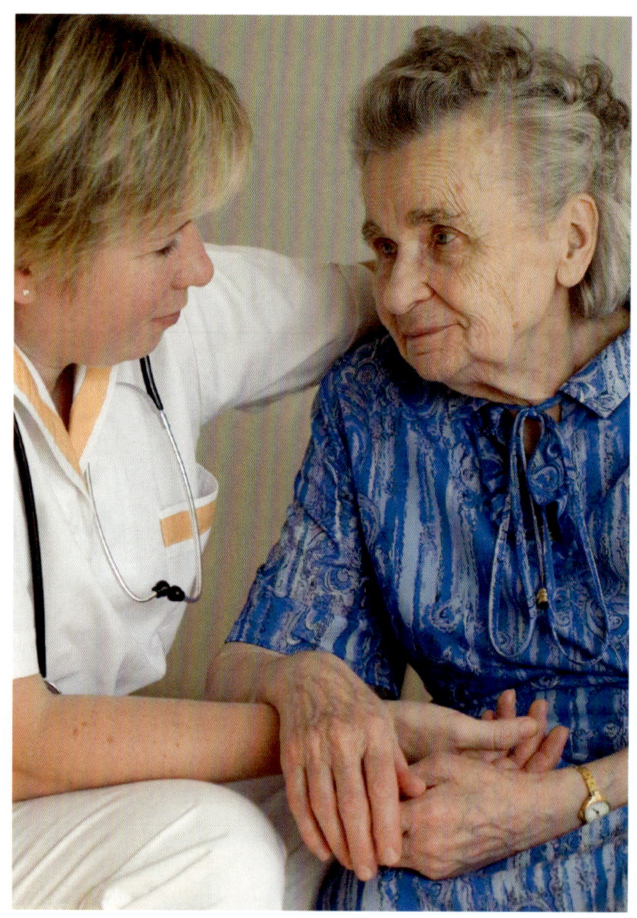

either at home or in institutions and need to ensure that care and professional staff and visitors are not perpetrating maltreatment by providing adequate training, resources and governance structures.

## 1.4 Why older people need special attention?

Older people may be vulnerable to elder maltreatment in the home and in other settings. In old age, particularly in later life and nearing the end of life, people may develop ill health, become frail and be unable to independently undertake activities of daily living, increasing their dependence on others and hence their vulnerability to maltreatment. Older people therefore need some safeguards to protect their human rights (Box 1.1). The prevention of elder maltreatment and the protection of older people should therefore be key policy priorities. Older people should be regarded as respected members of society who are able to lead full lives and contribute to society. Further, for the older people who rely on other people to ensure that they get the best of care at home or in other settings, it is essential that this trust and expectation not be broken.

Societal attitudes of ageism and negative attitudes towards older people and stereotyping may devalue and marginalize older people. This may result in lower self-esteem and increase the likelihood of social exclusion and threaten people's ability to have a fulfilled life. Maltreatment worsens social isolation, thereby perpetuating a vicious cycle in which older people who are isolated are more likely to be maltreated. Further, elder

**Box 1.1. Why is elder maltreatment a health and social problem?**

Humanitarian – it causes great suffering to individuals or groups within a society.

Functional – it threatens the fabric of society.

Cost – it drains resources and requires societal investment.

Social justice – some older people are vulnerable and their rights should be protected.

Social norms – regarding behaviour and expectations.

Prevalence – overall, many people suffer from elder maltreatment, and special services and programmes are needed *(16)*.

Burden – a cause of premature death and disability.

Response – the health and care sectors are in the front line for prevention, detection and rehabilitation.

maltreatment is associated with extreme stress, confers an additional risk of death and further reduces survival *(16)*.

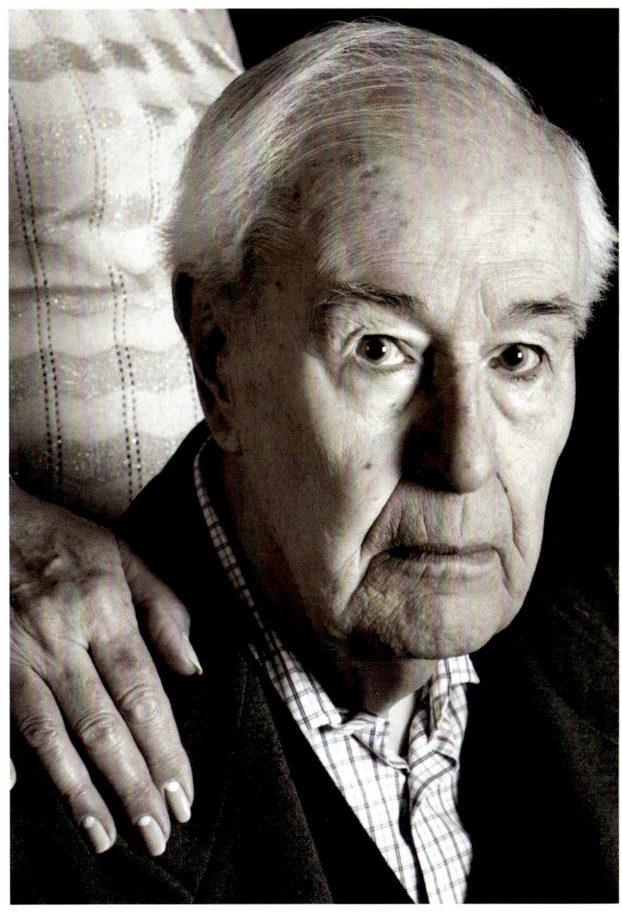

Across the globe, countries need to ensure that older people can live with dignity, integrity and independence and without maltreatment. The Madrid International Plan of Action on Ageing *(17)* sought to address the problem of social exclusion and called for initiatives to respond to the inequality, marginalization, deprivation and violence that many older people experience *(18)*. Older people who may be socially excluded based on their age, sex, income, education, social support network, health status and culture merit special attention, and focusing on their determinants of health may also promote their social inclusion *(18)*.

## 1.5 Does elder maltreatment have a social pattern?

The link between poverty, income inequality and the occurrence of elder maltreatment is an important question for all countries in the European Region. Little direct evidence indicates that elder maltreatment differs by socioeconomic status. This is unlike the situation for all-cause mortality, in which older people with lower education attainment have higher mortality rates *(19)*.

Among young people, both fatal and nonfatal interpersonal violence rates are several times higher in the most deprived sections of society than the most affluent sections, even in high-income countries *(20–23)*. This is also true for hospital admissions for violent assault among older people living in deprived areas, which are several times higher (11 times for men and 4 times for women) than among older residents of affluent neighbourhoods *(24)*. Nevertheless, similar to other causes of violence *(25)*, elder maltreatment probably has a social pattern. Of the few studies reporting this, one from the United Kingdom *(26)* reports a much higher prevalence among people who had been in routine or semi-routine occupations than among those who had been small employers or self-employed. A study from Turkey (27) found more than twice the prevalence of elder maltreatment if the educational level was primary school or lower versus secondary school or higher. In Israel, a higher educational level protected against verbal abuse *(28)*, and in a rural community in Finland, previous occupation as a farmer among women was associated with an increased prevalence of elder maltreatment *(29)*. Although there have been other community surveys, these have not properly examined the role of socioeconomic risk factors *(30–32)*. In a multicountry study of seven European countries, living in rented accommodation versus home ownership appeared to be associated with mental abuse, and having been a homemaker was associated with physical abuse *(7)*. Of interest, some studies report that having a higher educational level is associated with a greater likelihood of reporting maltreatment given the stigma associated with reporting it *(33)*. Better-designed studies are needed to improve the evidence base of the determinants of socioeconomic risk. Risk factors for elder maltreatment such as alcohol and drug dependence among perpetrators are linked to socioeconomic class and deprivation. Further, some studies have found social support networks to be protective *(34)*.

In many countries, many older people live in near poverty, leaving them with fewer resources to look after themselves and increasing their dependence on family and state support. The prevalence of poverty among people older than 65 years (defined as having less than 60% of the national median income) is very unequal across Europe. For the European Union (EU) countries, the prevalence is 4% in Hungary, 5% in Luxembourg and 7% in the Czech Republic but 51% in Latvia, 49% in Cyprus and 39% in Estonia *(35)*. The risk of poverty grows with older age and is much higher among women than men.

In the European Region, social determinants are important given the current economic recession and the evident decline of social support networks. This is of particular concern in the Commonwealth of Independent States (CIS)[3] countries, where the transition to market economies has been associated with reduced retirement incomes and fewer health and welfare services, resulting in greater hardship and more dependence on families *(36)*. There is renewed concern that the economic recession of 2008 and beyond will raise mortality from homicides and suicides *(37)*. High unemployment, rising income inequality, loss of social support networks and high alcohol consumption levels also contribute to exacerbating violence. These forces are eroding family, community and social networks that previously provided support to the older generations. Estimates from past mortality and unemployment patterns suggest that, in the EU countries, every 1% increase in unemployment has resulted in a 0.8% increase in homicide and suicide rates for all ages taken together. The effects are more marked for homicides in which older people are victims and seem to be worse in countries with less social protection and without active labour market programmes *(37)*.

## 1.6 How to overcome elder maltreatment

In recent decades, elder maltreatment has been recognized as a problem that should be tackled through coordinated public health action and an evidence-informed public health approach, similar to other forms of interpersonal violence *(1)*. The societal response has been inadequately developed in most countries so far. The health sector has a leading role to

3 The CIS consisted of Armenia, Azerbaijan, Belarus, Georgia, Kazakhstan, Kyrgyzstan, the Republic of Moldova, the Russian Federation, Tajikistan, Turkmenistan, Ukraine and Uzbekistan when the data were collected.

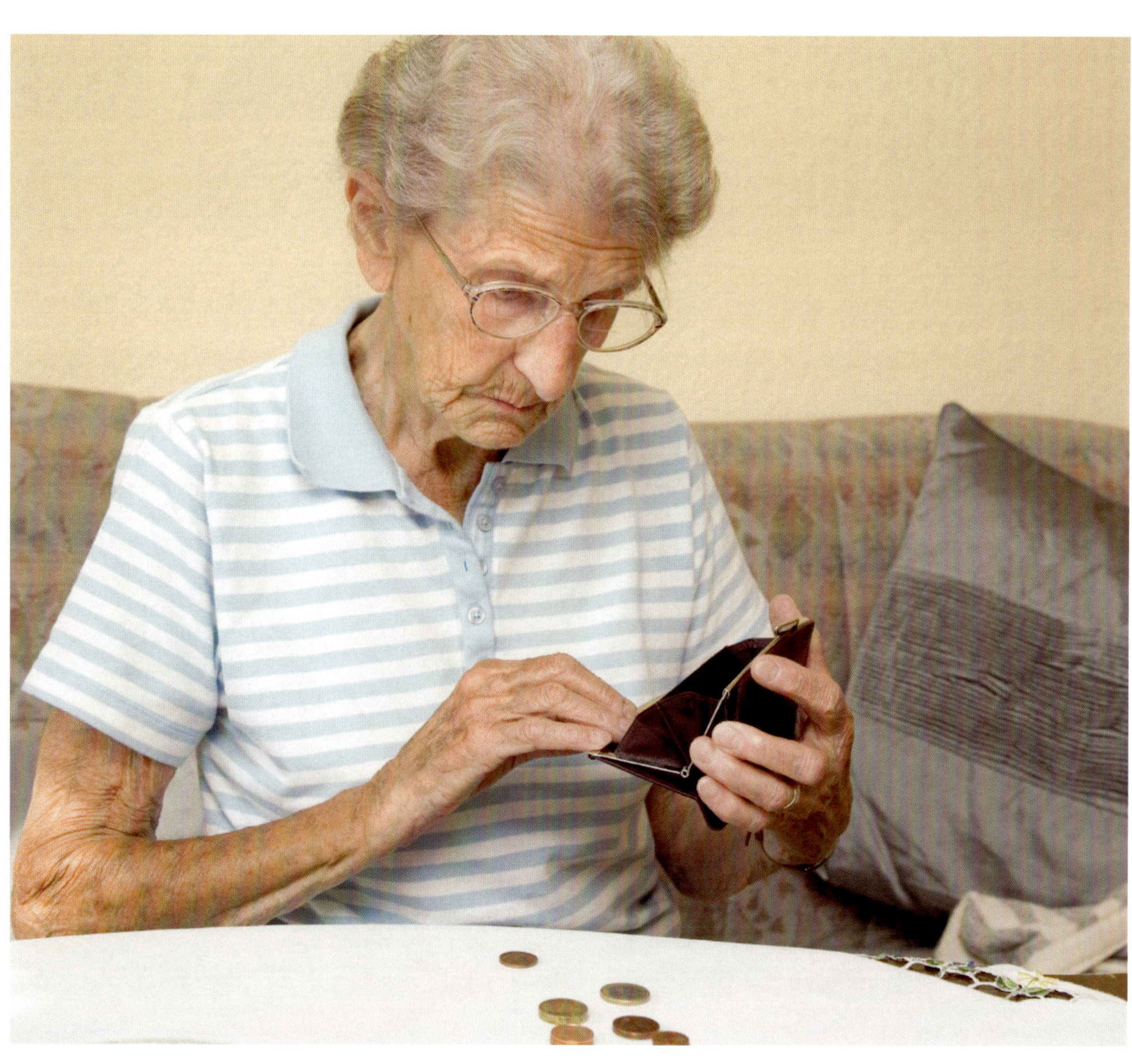

play in documenting the burden, identifying risk factors, distilling the evidence of what works and coordinating an intersectoral public health response to the problem *(1,38–41)*. Key among these actions is multidisciplinary research to quantify the extent, causes, costs and effects of elder maltreatment and the action needed for prevention *(42)*. This is a particular challenge for elder maltreatment, since there has been little evidence-informed documentation, especially of interventions for primary prevention.

Current thinking contests the notion that violence is an inevitable part of human life and shows that much violence can be predicted and is preventable *(1)*. Similar to other forms of violence, elder maltreatment results from complex interaction among many factors at the individual, relationship, community and societal levels. The ecological model is useful for considering risks and is valuable for understanding the types of programmes that need to be targeted at the different levels (Fig. 1.1) *(1,43,44)*. The following chapters of this report use this model extensively.

Successful responses to violence involve a public health approach that accounts for the size of the problem, the risk factors and the evidence base of what works and then implements these on a wider scale *(45)*. Greater emphasis is needed in undertaking this evidence-informed approach in tackling the problem of elder maltreatment. Investing in safety is a societal responsibility involving various sectors in providing safe physical and social environments for older people. A life-course approach is increasing acknowledged as being needed to prevent interpersonal violence in later life *(1,42,46)*. Implementation of evidence-informed approaches would reduce much pain and suffering and save many lives. Since few studies have assessed the effectiveness of interventions for preventing elder maltreatment, this implies a need for more outcome research and using an evaluative framework in implementing preventive programmes. This report critically reviews the existing evidence on preventing elder maltreatment.

## 1.7 What types of pressure will countries feel with an ageing population?

Most countries in the European Region have experienced improved health and increased life expectancy in the past two decades, although in some CIS countries this has declined. Life expectancy in the Region is generally higher among women than men by several years (Fig. 1.2), and since women outlive men, the proportion of older women among older people is higher than that of men, and this increases at older age.

Most but not all of this time is spent in good health. The healthy life expectancy (HALE) at birth represents the average number of years that a person could expect to live in "good health" and is shown in Annex 2, Fig. 1. The years of relatively poor health are when older people may be more vulnerable to maltreatment because of greater dependence or disability.

The population of the WHO European Region is ageing rapidly. Most countries have witnessed declines in fertility and increases in life expectancy, including among older age groups *(48,49)*. These trends are expected to continue in the European Region, and the proportion of people 65 years and older is predicted to grow from 14% in 2010 to 25% in 2050 (Fig. 1.3, Box 1.2). This is predicted to be 29% for the EU in 2050 and 21% for the CIS. By 2050, one third of the population of the European Region will be 60 years and older *(50)*.

As a consequence, pensions will have to be paid for a longer time and, since not all the years gained are likely to be lived in optimum health, more resources will be needed to provide health and social care. Having a higher proportion of the population that is dependent compared with those of working age (15–64 years) will be a source of extra strain on economic, social and family structures (Annex 2, Fig. 2). To ease the economic pressure, some countries are responding to the extra longevity by deferring the age at which people can

**Fig. 1.1. An ecological framework on levels of intervention against elder maltreatment**

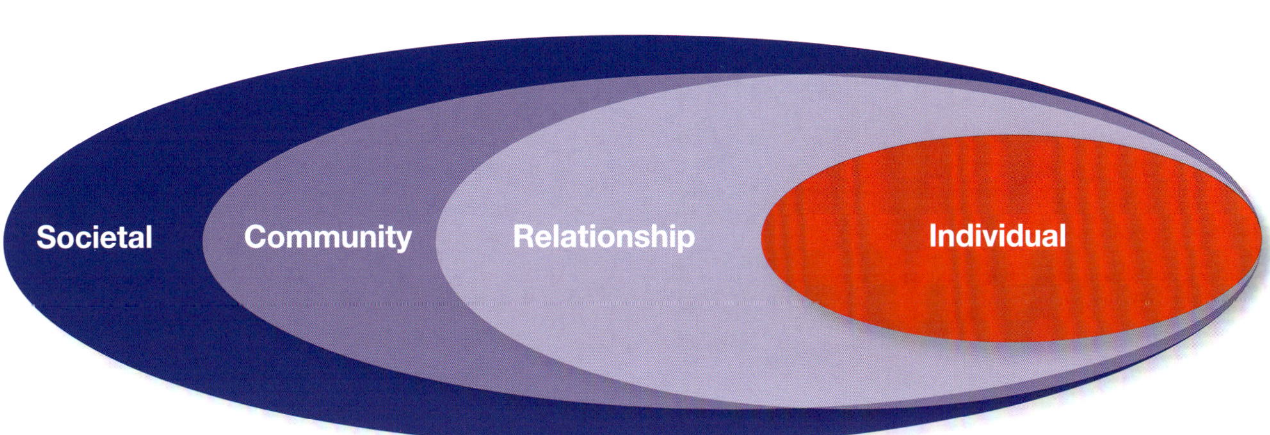


*Sources:* Krug et al. *(1)* and Butchart et al. *(42)*, based on Bronfenbrenner *(44)*.

**Fig. 1.2. Life expectancy at birth for males and females for countries in the WHO European Region, 2008 (or most recent year)**

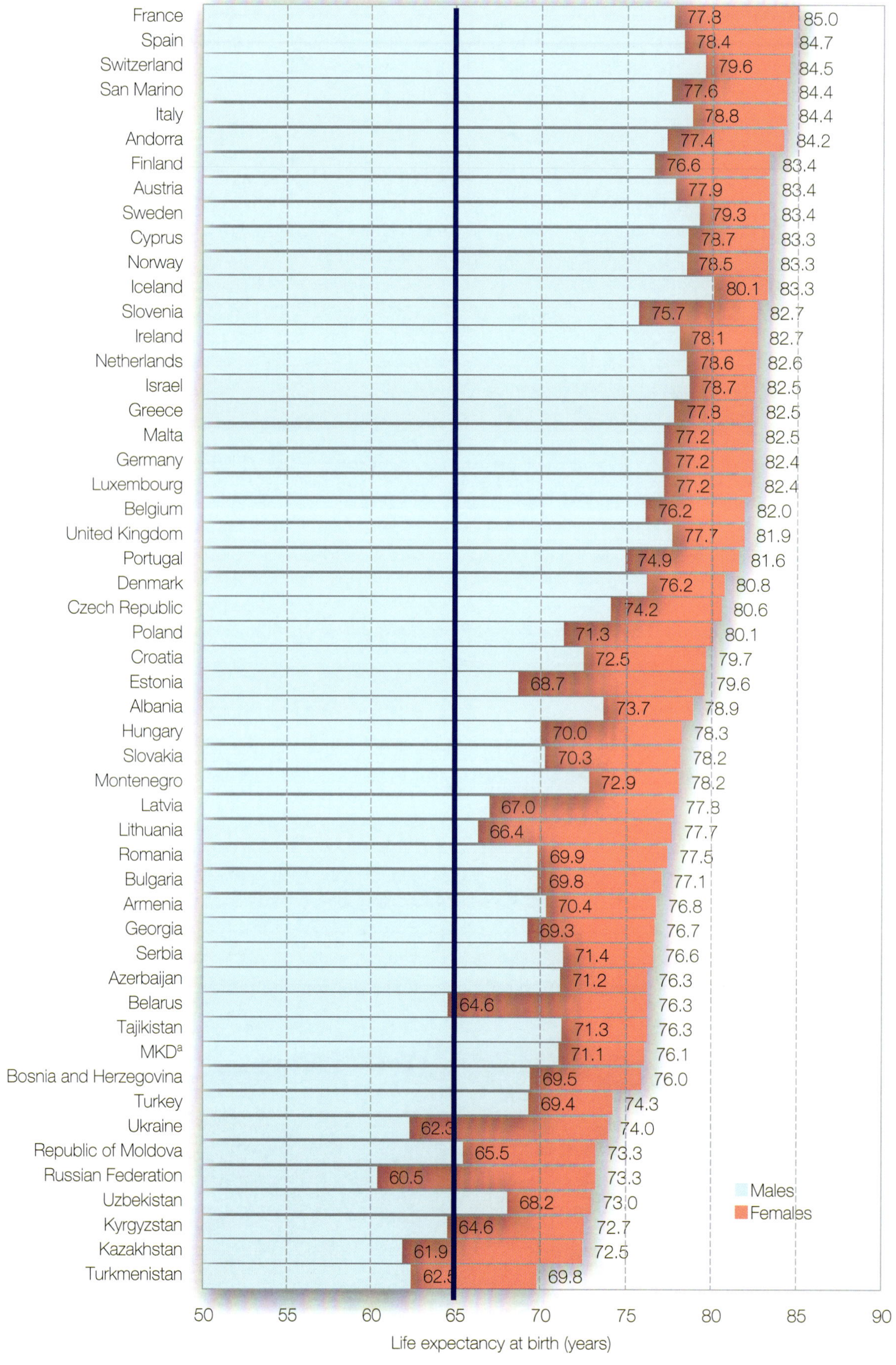


[a] MKD stands for the former Yugoslav Republic of Macedonia; it is an abbreviation of the International Organization for Standardization (ISO), not WHO.
*Source:* European Health for All mortality database *(47)*.

**Fig. 1.3. Percentage of the population 65 years and older in the WHO European Region, EU and CIS**

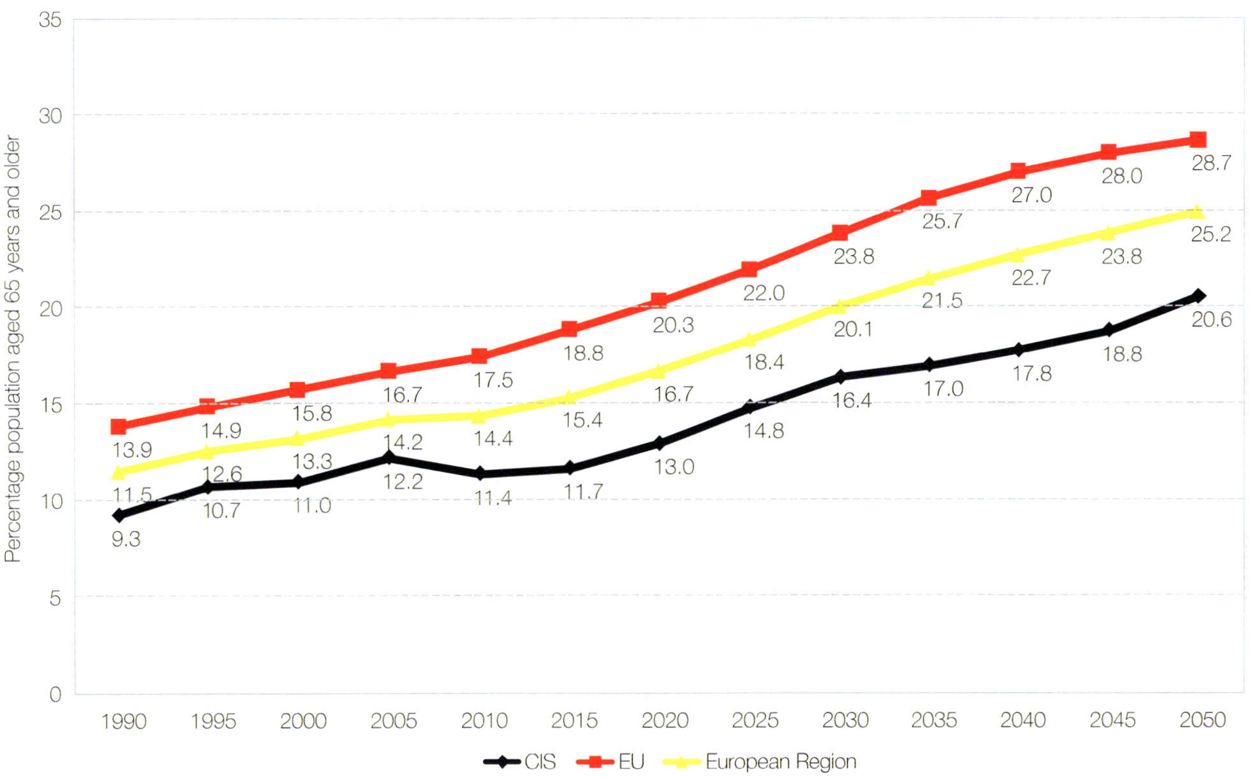


*Source:* United Nations, Department of Economic and Social Affairs, Population Division *(50)*.

**Box 1.2. Challenges of population ageing in the European Region**

Strains on pensions and social security systems.

Increasing demands for health and social care.

Greater demands made on family caregivers.

A greater need for a trained health and care workforce.

Meeting the demand for long-term care, particularly in supporting people with dementia and multiple problems.

Preserving the rights for older people that are denied by ageism.

Retaining and strengthening social cohesion and solidarity across generations.

obtain public retirement benefits to 68 years, such as in the United Kingdom, although there are calls to raise this to 70 years by 2040 *(51)*. The greater economic and social pressure may also influence the likelihood of elder maltreatment. For many people, greater longevity is also associated with a longer period of frailty, impaired activities of daily living and ill health, putting extra pressure on family and social welfare support *(52)*. The proportion of the population requiring care by family caregivers is likely to increase, and it has been suggested that the period of transition into caregiving needs to be given particular attention *(28)*. Social cohesion across generations will need to be strengthened in all countries to meet this challenge.

The proportion of the population aged 65 years and older that receives formal (not family) long-term care services either at home or in care settings ranges from 1% in Azerbaijan to 30% in Iceland, and the average for the EU is 11% (Fig. 1.4). Much of this variation results from national health and welfare policies and resources. Older people receiving formal care are more vulnerable to maltreatment in these settings.

### 1.8 What are the global and regional policy dimensions linked to preventing elder maltreatment?

Conventions and charters adopted by Member States in the European Region enshrine the principles of equity, solidarity and protecting the rights of citizens. The Tallinn Charter: Health Systems for Health and Wealth *(54)* emphasizes that health systems have a central role in promoting equity, calling for greater attention to the needs of poor and vulnerable people. The Universal Declaration of Human Rights can be interpreted as highlighting social responsibility to protect citizens, including those who are vulnerable such as older people, to provide them with appropriate support and

**Fig. 1.4. Percentage of the population aged 65 years and older that receives formal long-term care services either at home or in institutions in selected countries, WHO European Region**

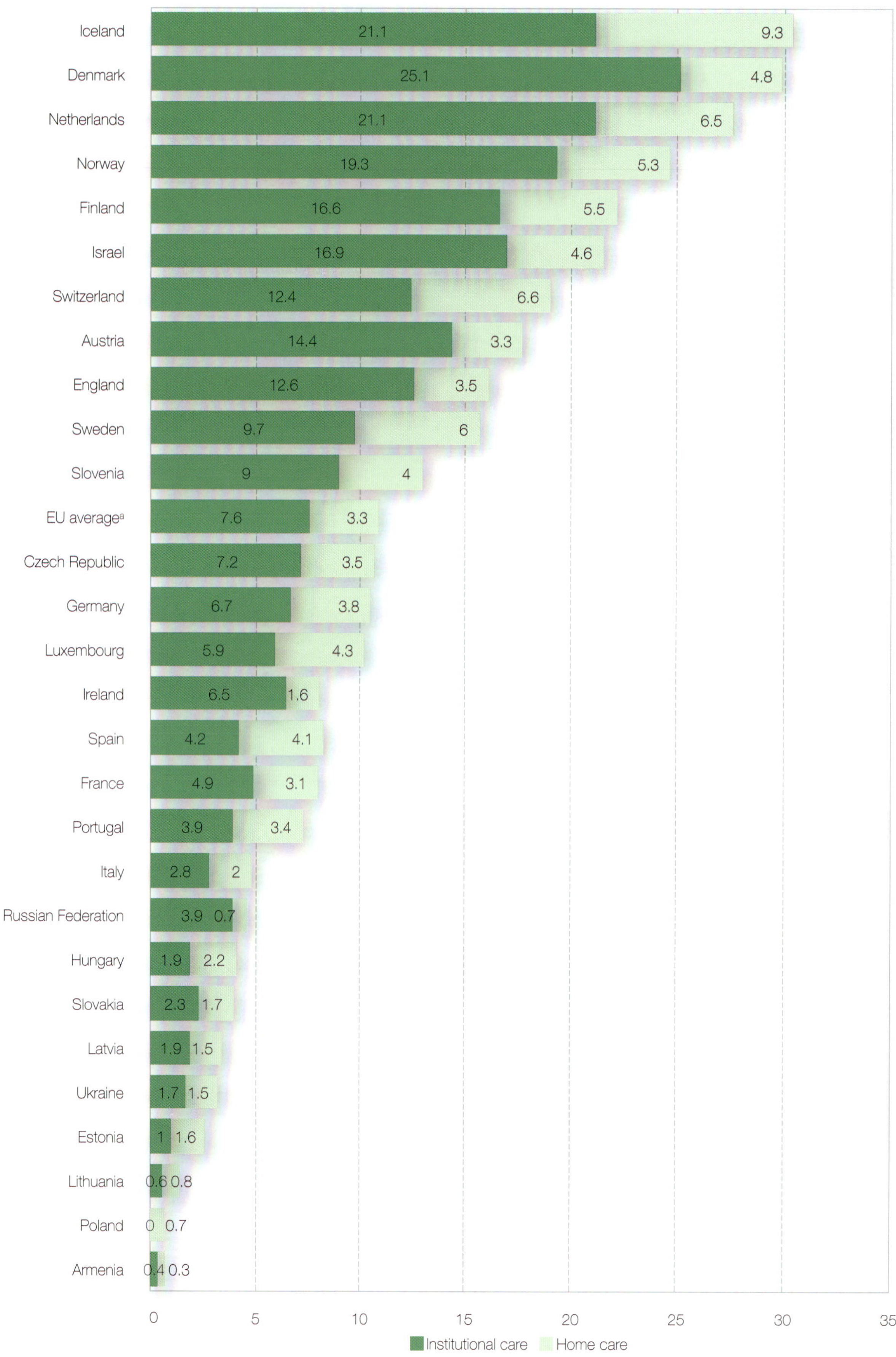


[a] Unweighted average of available data from EU countries for various years.
*Source:* Huber et al. *(53)*.

services and promote their right to a safe environment that is free from violence. More recently, the Second United Nations World Assembly on Ageing recognized the special needs of older people *(17)*, and this led to the Toronto Declaration on the Global Prevention of Elder Abuse *(55)*. This call for action focuses on legal frameworks, a multisectoral plan of action, social marketing and promoting the role of primary health care workers in the front line of prevention. In recognition of the global demographic shift, the Madrid International Plan of Action on Ageing *(17)* promotes international collaboration to take advantage of the opportunities and to respond to the challenges of an ageing population. These strongly emphasize healthy and active ageing and empowering and protecting older people to defend their right to a safe environment. A recent review of the policy response by governments has shown that much more action is needed *(2, 40)*. The report of the Commission on Social Determinants of Health *(56)* emphasizes that the unequal distribution of power, income, goods and services leads to inequity in health within and between countries and highlights older people as a group at higher risk. Many of the risk factors for violence and maltreatment are linked to these structural determinants and conditions of daily living in societies. Unsafe neighbourhoods, high unemployment, misuse of alcohol and drugs, diminishing social networks and poor access to health and social services predispose older people to maltreatment. The current report strongly makes the case for tackling these social determinants of health as part of a life-course approach to preventing maltreatment.

**Key messages**

The prevalence of elder maltreatment in the community is high.

If unchecked, elder maltreatment leads to reduced survival and poorer quality of life.

The numbers of people affected by elder maltreatment are likely to increase with the ageing of the population.

Action therefore needs to be taken to halt this potential increase.

Preventing elder maltreatment is an issue of human rights and social solidarity.

Social inclusion and cross-generational cohesion needs to be strengthened.

The lack of good research evidence about how to prevent elder maltreatment is a challenge.

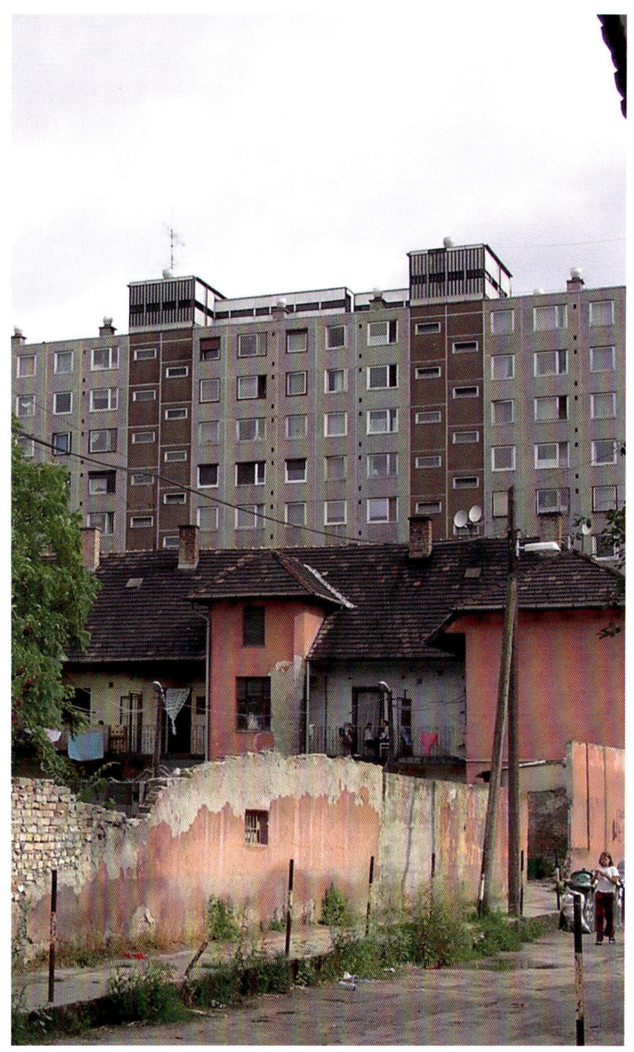

## 1.9 References


1. Krug E et al., eds. *World report on violence and health*. Geneva, World Health Organization, 2002 (http://www.who.int/violence_injury_prevention/violence/world_report/en, accessed 9 May 2011).
2. Podnieks E et al. WorldView Environmental Scan on Elder Abuse. *Journal of Elder Abuse and Neglect*, 2010, 22:164–179.
3. Baker AA. Granny bashing. *Modern Geriatrics*, 1975, 5:20–24.
4. Burston GR. "Granny bashing". *British Medical Journal*, 1975, 3:352.
5. Ageing [web site]. Geneva, World Health Organization, 2011 (http://www.who.int/topics/ageing/en, accessed 9 May 2011).
6. *Understanding elder maltreatment*. Atlanta, United States Centers for Disease Control and Prevention, 2010 (http://www.cdc.gov/violenceprevention/pdf/em-factsheet-a.pdf, accessed 9 May 2011).
7. Soares JJF et al. *Abuse and health in Europe*. Kaunas, Lithuanian University of Health Sciences Press, 2010.
8. Cooper C, Selwood A, Livingston G. The prevalence of elder abuse and neglect: a systematic review. *Age and Aging*, 2008, 37:151–160.

9. Shields LBE, Hunsaker DM, Hunsaker JC. Abuse and neglect: a ten year review of mortality and morbidity in our elders in a large metropolitan area. *Journal of Forensic Sciences*, 2004, 49:122–127.

10. Ahmad M, Lachs MS. Elder abuse and neglect: what physicians can and should do. *Cleveland Clinic Journal of Medicine*, 2002, 69:801–808.

11. Rovi S et al. Mapping the elder mistreatment iceberg: U.S. hospitalizations with elder abuse and neglect diagnoses. *Journal of Elder Abuse and Neglect*, 2009, 21:346–359.

12. Lachs MS, Pillemer K. Abuse and neglect of elderly persons. *New England Journal of Medicine*, 1995, 332:437–443.

13. *The global burden of disease: 2004 update*. Geneva, World Health Organization, 2008 (http://www.who.int/healthinfo/global_burden_disease/2004_report_update/en/index.html, accessed 9 May 2011).

14. Iborra I, ed. *Violencia contra personas mayores [Violence against older people]*. Barcelona, Editorial Ariel, 2005 (Colección Estudios sobre Violencia, No. 11).

15. Collins KA, Presnell SE. Elder homicide. A 20-year study. American Journal of Forensic Medicine and Pathology, 2006, 27:183–187.

16. Lachs MS et al. The mortality of elder maltreatment. *Journal of the American Medical Association*, 1998, 280:428–432.

17. *Report of the Second World Assembly on Ageing, Madrid, 8–12 April 2002*. New York, United Nations, 2002 (http://daccess-dds-ny.un.org/doc/UNDOC/GEN/N02/397/51/PDF/N0239751.pdf?OpenElement, accessed 9 May 2011).

18. Podnieks E. Social inclusion: an interplay of the determinants of health – new insights into elder abuse. *Journal of Gerontology and Social Work*, 2006, 46(3–4):57–79.

19. Huisman M et al. Socioeconomic inequalities in mortality among elderly people in 11 European populations. *Journal of Epidemiology and Community Health*, 2004, 58:468–475.

20. Leyland AH, Dundas R. The social patterning of deaths due to assault in Scotland, 1980–2005: a population based study *Journal of Epidemiology and Community Health*, 2010, 64:432–439.

21. Bellis MA et al. Contribution of violence to health inequalities in England: demographics and trends in emergency hospital admissions for assault. *Journal of Epidemiology and Community Health*, 2008, 62:1064–1071.

22. Roberts I, Power C. Does the decline in child injury mortality vary by social class? A comparison of class specific mortality in 1981 and 1991. *British Medical Journal*, 1996, 313:784–786.

23. Sethi D et al. *European report on preventing violence and knife crime among young people*. Copenhagen, WHO Regional Office for Europe, 2010 (http://www.euro.who.int/__data/assets/pdf_file/0012/121314/E94277.pdf, accessed 9 May 2011).

24. Bellis MA et al. National five-year examination of inequalities and trends in emergency hospital admission for violence across England. *Injury Prevention*, doi:10.1136/ip.2010.030486.

25. Wilkinson RG, Kawachi I, Kennedy BP. Mortality, the social environment, crime and violence. *Sociology of Health and Illness*, 1998, 20:578–597.

26. Biggs S et al. Mistreatment of the older people in the United Kingdom: findings from the first National Prevalence Study. *Journal of Elder Abuse and Neglect*, 2009, 21:1–14.

27. Kissal A, Beser A. Elder abuse and neglect in a population offering care by a primary health care center in Izmir, Turkey. *Social Work in Health Care*, 2011, 50:158–175.

28. Lowenstein A et al. Is elder abuse and neglect a social phenomenon? Data from the first national prevalence survey in Israel. *Journal of Elder Abuse and Neglect*, 2009, 21:253–277.

29. Kivela SL et al. Abuse in old age – epidemiological data from Finland. *Journal of Elder Abuse and Neglect*, 1992, 4:1–18.

30. Comijs HC et al. Psychological distress in victims of elder mistreatment: the effects of social support and coping. *Journal of Gerontology Series B – Psychological Sciences and Social Sciences*, 1999, 54:240–245.

31. Pillimer K, Finkelhor D. The prevalence of elder abuse: a random sample survey. *The Gerontologist*, 1988, 28:51–57.

32. Podnieks E. National survey on abuse of the elderly in Canada. *Journal of Elder Abuse and Neglect*, 1992:5–58.

33. Cohen M et al. Elder abuse: disparities between older people's disclosure of abuse, evident signs of abuse, and high risk of abuse. *Journal of the American Geriatric Society*, 2007, 55:1224–1230.

34. Dong XQ, Simon MA. Is greater social support a protective factor against elder maltreatment? *Gerontology*, 2008, 54:381–388.

35. Zaidi A. *Poverty risks for older people in EU countries – an update*. Vienna, European Centre for Social Welfare Policy and Research, 2010.

36. McKee M et al. Health policy-making in central and eastern Europe: why has there been so little action on injuries? *Health Policy and Planning*, 2000, 15:263–269.

37. Stuckler D et al. The public health effect of economic crises and alternative policy responses in Europe: an empirical analysis. *Lancet*, 2009, 374:315–323.

38. Sethi D et al. *Injuries and violence in Europe: why they matter and what can be done*. Copenhagen, WHO Regional Office for Europe, 2006 (http://www.euro.who.int/__data/assets/pdf_file/0007/98404/E87321.pdf, accessed 9 May 2011).

39. Sethi D et al. Reducing inequalities from injuries in Europe. *Lancet*, 2006, 368:2243–2250.

40. Sethi D et al. *Preventing injuries in Europe: from international collaboration to local implementation*. Copenhagen, WHO Regional Office for Europe, 2010 (http://www.euro.who.int/en/what-we-publish/abstracts/preventing-injuries-in-europe-from-international-collaboration-to-local-implementation, accessed 9 May 2011).

41. *World Health Assembly resolution WHA56.24 on implementing the recommendations of the* World report on violence and health. Geneva, World Health Organization, 2003 (http://whqlibdoc.who.int/wha/2003/WHA56_24.pdf, accessed 9 May 2011).

42. Butchart A et al. *Preventing violence. A guide to implementing the recommendations of the* World report on violence and health. Geneva, World Health Organization, 2004 (http://www.who.int/violence_injury_prevention/media/news/08_09_2004/en/index.html, accessed 9 May 2011).

43. Mercy JA et al. Public health policy for preventing violence. *Health Affairs*, 1993, 12:4.

44. Bronfenbrenner U. *The ecology of human development*. Cambridge, Harvard University Press, 1979.

45. *Preventing injuries and violence: a guide for ministries of health*. Geneva, World Health Organization, 2007 (http://www.who.int/violence_injury_prevention/publications/injury_policy_planning/prevention_moh/en/index.html, accessed 9 May 2011).

46. *Violence prevention: the evidence*. Geneva, World Health Organization, 2010 (http://www.who.int/violence_injury_prevention/violence/4th_milestones_meeting/publications/en/index.html, accessed 9 May 2011).

47. European Health for All mortality database [online database]. Copenhagen, WHO Regional Office for Europe, 2010 (http://www.euro.who.int/hfadb, accesed 9 May 2011).

48. Zaidi A. *Features and challenges of population aging: the European perspective*. Vienna, European Centre for Social Welfare Policy and Research, 2008.

49. Kinsella K. Demographic dimensions of global aging. *Journal of Family Issues*, 2000, 21:541–558.

50. Population Database [online database]. New York, United Nations, Department of Economic and Social Affairs, Population Division, 2010 (http://esa.un.org/unpd/wpp/unpp/panel_population.htm, accessed 9 May 2011).

51. 70 or bust. Current plans to raise the retirement age are not bold enough. *The Economist*, 2011, 9 April:13.

52. Lafortune G et al. *Trends in severe disability among elderly people: assessing the evidence from 12 OECD countries and future implications*. Paris, Organisation for Economic Co-operation and Development, 2007 (OECD Health Working Papers No. 26).

53. Huber M et al. *Facts and figures on long-term care. Europe and North America*. Vienna, European Centre for Social Welfare Policy and Research, in press.

54. *The Tallinn Charter: Health Systems for Health and Wealth*. Copenhagen, WHO Regional Office for Europe, 2008 (http://www.euro.who.int/__data/assets/pdf_file/0008/886613/E91438.pdf, accessed 9 May 2011).

55. *The Toronto Declaration on the Global Prevention of Elder Abuse*. Geneva, World Health Organization, 2002 (http://www.who.int/ageing/projects/elder_abuse/en/index.html, accessed 9 May 2011).

56. Commission on Social Determinants of Health. *Closing the gap in a generation: health equity through action on the social determinants of health. Final report of the Commission on Social Determinants of Health*. Geneva, World Health Organization, 2008 (http://www.who.int/social_determinants/resources/gkn_lee_al.pdf, accessed 9 May 2011).

# 2. Scale of the problem

This chapter uses various data sources to describe elder maltreatment. It has two main sections. The first section addresses homicides with older people as victims, and the second section focuses on information from surveys of elder maltreatment in the community and in other settings. Whereas data on homicide deaths among older people are reliable and complete in the European Region, there is little routine information on deaths that are attributable to elder maltreatment, and this information needs to be estimated. Similarly, other routine sources of data such as hospital admission and emergency department data and police data are less than complete and depend on elder maltreatment being reported to the police or coming to the attention of the health or care sector, and they are considered to be grossly underreported *(1,2)*. The second section reports on findings mainly from the European literature covering surveys of elder maltreatment. Population surveys, asking people whether they have been victims or perpetrators, offer a more complete data set, although these may be influenced by responder bias and survey methods.

**Key facts**

About 8300 people aged 60 years and older die from homicide annually in the WHO European Region.

Nine of ten homicide deaths among older people are in low- and middle-income countries.

Elder maltreatment causes an estimated 2500 (30%) of these.

The prevalence of elder maltreatment in the previous year in the community is high in the Region:

- 2.7% have experienced physical abuse – equivalent to 4 million older people;
- 0.7% have experienced sexual abuse – equivalent to 1 million older people;
- 19.4% have experienced mental abuse – equivalent to 29 million older people; and
- 3.8% have experienced financial abuse – equivalent to 6 million older people.

The prevalence increases among people with disabilities, cognitive impairment and dependence.

## 2.1 Proportion of homicide deaths among older people attributable to elder maltreatment

Estimates from the literature suggest that a family member perpetrates about 30% of homicide deaths among older people (Table 2.1) *(3)*. This is corroborated by studies from the United States of America showing similar proportions *(4,5)*. Based on this, elder maltreatment may cause an estimated 30% of the homicide deaths reported in routine databases because they have been committed by a family member.[4] This is likely to be an underestimate, as it would exclude elder maltreatment committed by non-family caregivers. Further, the intent of many deaths is undetermined, and many cases of elder maltreatment may also be undetected. There may well be great variation between countries. Despite these limitations, these data are the best available (Annex 1).

In cases of deaths from injury, where intent is not determined, these are recorded as being of undetermined intent. There are an estimated 10 800 injury deaths of undetermined intent annually among people aged 60 years and older in the WHO European Region, and a proportion of these may be attributed to elder maltreatment (estimated from the Global Burden of Disease project *(6)* and European detailed mortality database). A proportion of these may represent cases of homicide and elder maltreatment that have not been properly ascertained. Death certification and the case detection of elder maltreatment need to be improved.

## 2.2 Mortality and burden of injuries from interpersonal violence

In the European Region, 8300 people aged 60 years and older die from interpersonal violence annually. Men account for 52% of these deaths *(6)*. Data show that 4% of all injury deaths in older people are due to interpersonal violence (Fig. 2.1). There is a similar pattern for the burden of injuries, and 4% of the burden of injuries is attributable to interpersonal violence[5] (see Annex 2, Fig. 3).

### *2.2.1 Homicide rates by age and sex*

Mortality rates from homicide are higher among men than among women at all ages, except people aged 80 years and older. Among older people, the rates are higher among men aged 60–69 years (7.8 per 100 000) and women aged 70–79 years (4.5 per 100 000) (Fig. 2.2).

[4] Whereas an assumption is made here that the proportion of 30% might apply to all countries in the Region, countries and cultures could vary considerably. Similarly, not all cases of homicide committed by family members might be consistent with the definition of elder maltreatment. Nevertheless, these are the best data available. See Annex 3.

[5] The burden of injuries is measured in disability-adjusted life-years (DALYs). One DALY is a composite measure of one year of life lost due to premature mortality and lived with disability.

**Table 2.1. Percentage of homicides among people aged 60 years and older committed by family members in selected countries, WHO European Region, 2000–2002**

| Country | 2000 | 2001 | 2002 | Average |
|---|---|---|---|---|
| Finland | | 27.3 | | 27.3 |
| Hungary | 31.0 | 30.8 | 31.1 | 30.9 |
| Iceland | 100.0 | 0.0 | 0.0 | 33.3 |
| Ireland | 50.0 | 20.0 | | 35.0 |
| Italy | 34.0 | 37.4 | 53.8 | 41.7 |
| Netherlands | 0.0 | 0.0 | 6.7 | 2.2 |
| Spain | 21.7 | 33.9 | 38.6 | 31.4 |
| United Kingdom | 30.1 | 29.7 | 26.7 | 28.8 |
| Average | 38.1 | 22.4 | 13.4 | 28.8 |

*Source:* Iborra *(3)*.

**Fig. 2.1. Distribution of deaths from various causes of unintentional and intentional injuries among people aged 60 years and older in the WHO European Region**

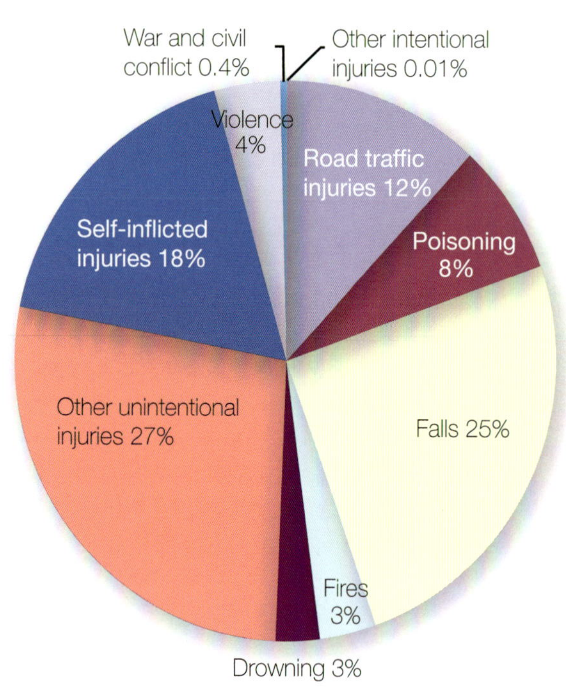


*Source*: *The global burden of disease: 2004 update (6).*

## 2.2.2 Inequality in homicide rates among older people in the European Region

The numbers of interpersonal violence deaths among people aged 60 years and older are highest in the low- and middle-income countries[6] in the European Region, where 9 of 10 deaths occur (7500 deaths). This percentage is similar for both sexes (90% among men and 91% among women).

There is a large gradient between high-income countries and low- and middle-income countries (Table 2.2). Homicide rates among people aged 60 years and older in low- and middle-income countries are 12 times higher than in high-income countries for both sexes: 13 times higher for men and 11 times higher for women.

Some countries in western Europe have the lowest homicide rates among people aged 60 years and older, and countries in the eastern part of the European Region have the highest rates. Within the EU, the Baltic countries have the highest rates. The homicide rates in the country with the highest (Russian Federation) and the lowest rates (United Kingdom) differ by 103-fold (122-fold among men and 95-fold among women) (Fig. 2.3). The mortality rate ratio among men versus women is 1.6 in the Region as a whole: 1.8 in low- and middle-income countries and 1.5 in high-income countries (Table 2.2). If all countries of the European Region had the same homicide rates as the country with the lowest rate, 96.7% of the deaths could potentially be avoided (8025 deaths every year).

## 2.2.3 Methods of homicide among older people

Data are available for 37 countries on the methods used to commit homicide among older people (see description on modes in Annex 1, Table 2). When taken together, most homicides are carried out as assaults with sharp objects (25%), followed by the use of bodily force (16%), firearms (14%), blunt objects (13%) and those due to hanging, strangulation and drowning (11%) (Fig. 2.4). However, the coding of deaths is incomplete, and 18% of deaths are

[6] Low- and middle-income countries: defined by World Bank definition 2001 (see Table 3 in Annex 1).

**Fig. 2.2. Homicide rates by age and sex in the WHO European Region, 2004**

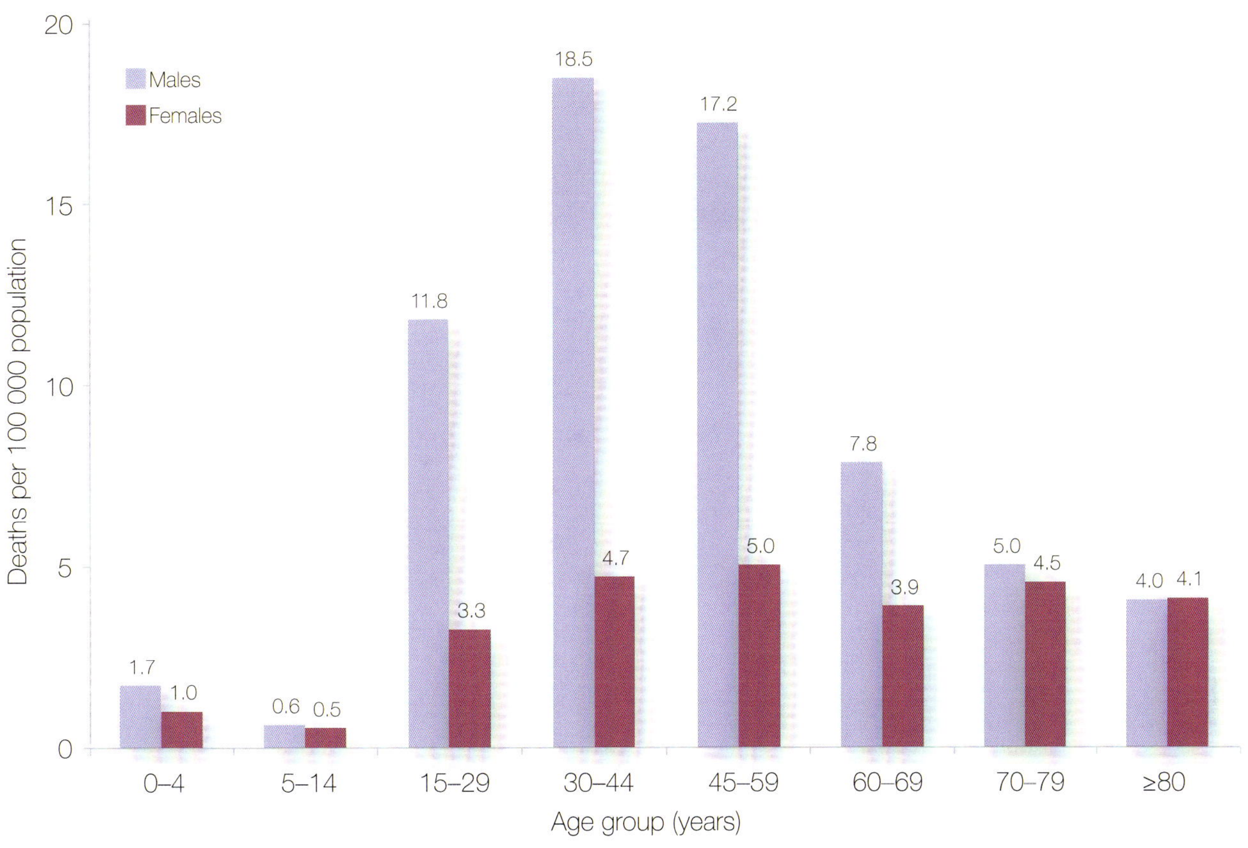


*Source: The global burden of disease: 2004 update (6).*

classified as having unspecified causes, with only 1% resulting from neglect. The countries in the Region vary greatly, and this is described for countries for which data are available (see Annex 2, Fig. 4).

### *2.2.4 Changes in homicide rates among older people over time*

Not only is there great diversity in the Region, but there are also rapid changes over time. Homicide rates among people aged 65 years and older peaked in the mid-1990s, followed by another peak in 2003. Although there has been a downward trend since then, homicide rates in the CIS countries still remain about 16 times higher than those in the EU (Fig. 2.5). Many countries are undergoing economic, political and social transition, and the forces of globalization are exerting material and social stress in many countries. These forces are eroding the family, community and social networks that previously provided support to the older generations. Low- and middle-income countries in the Region have undergone the most rapid changes politically in the transition to market economies. High unemployment, rising income inequality, loss of social support networks and high alcohol consumption have been proposed as causes of these peaks *(9)*.

**Table 2.2. Homicide rates and rate ratios per 100 000 population among people aged 60 years and older in low- and middle-income countries and high-income countries in the WHO European Region, 2004**

| | Men | Women | Both sexes | Rate ratio men/women |
|---|---|---|---|---|
| Low- and middle-income countries | 13.9 | 7.9 | 10.4 | 1.8 |
| High-income countries | 1.1 | 0.7 | 0.9 | 1.5 |
| All countries | 6.5 | 4.1 | 5.1 | 1.6 |
| Rate ratio between low- and middle-income countries and high-income countries | 12.9 | 11.4 | 12.0 | |

*Source: The global burden of disease: 2004 update (6).*

Fig. 2.3. Homicide rates per 100 000 people aged 60 years and older in the WHO European Region (average for 2004–2006 or last available 3 years)
Russian Federation 18.3
Kazakhstan 12.3
Kyrgyzstan 11.8
Belarus 10.7
Republic of Moldova 9.1
Ukraine 8.5
Latvia 7.9
Lithuania 7.6
Estonia 7.3
Albania 4.6
MKD[a] 4.5
Georgia 4.4
Uzbekistan 3.8
Romania 3.2
Bulgaria 2.7
Serbia 2.6
Hungary 2.3
Israel 2.1
Armenia 2.0
Slovakia 1.9
Belgium 1.8
Poland 1.7
Azerbaijan 1.5
Finland 1.5
Croatia 1.4
Luxembourg 1.4
Cyprus 1.4
Portugal 1.3
Greece 1.1
Malta 1.0
Spain 0.8
Sweden 0.8
Slovenia 0.7
Italy 0.7
Norway 0.7
Austria 0.7
Czech Republic 0.6
France 0.6
Denmark 0.5
Germany 0.5
Switzerland 0.5
Netherlands 0.5
Ireland 0.4
United Kingdom 0.2
0
2
4
6
8
10
12
14
16
18
20
Low- and middle-income countries
High-income countries

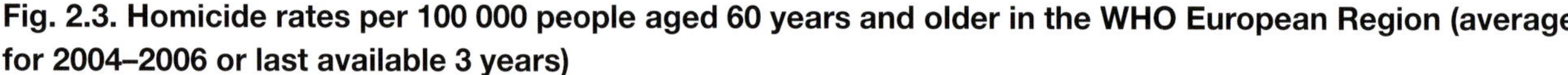

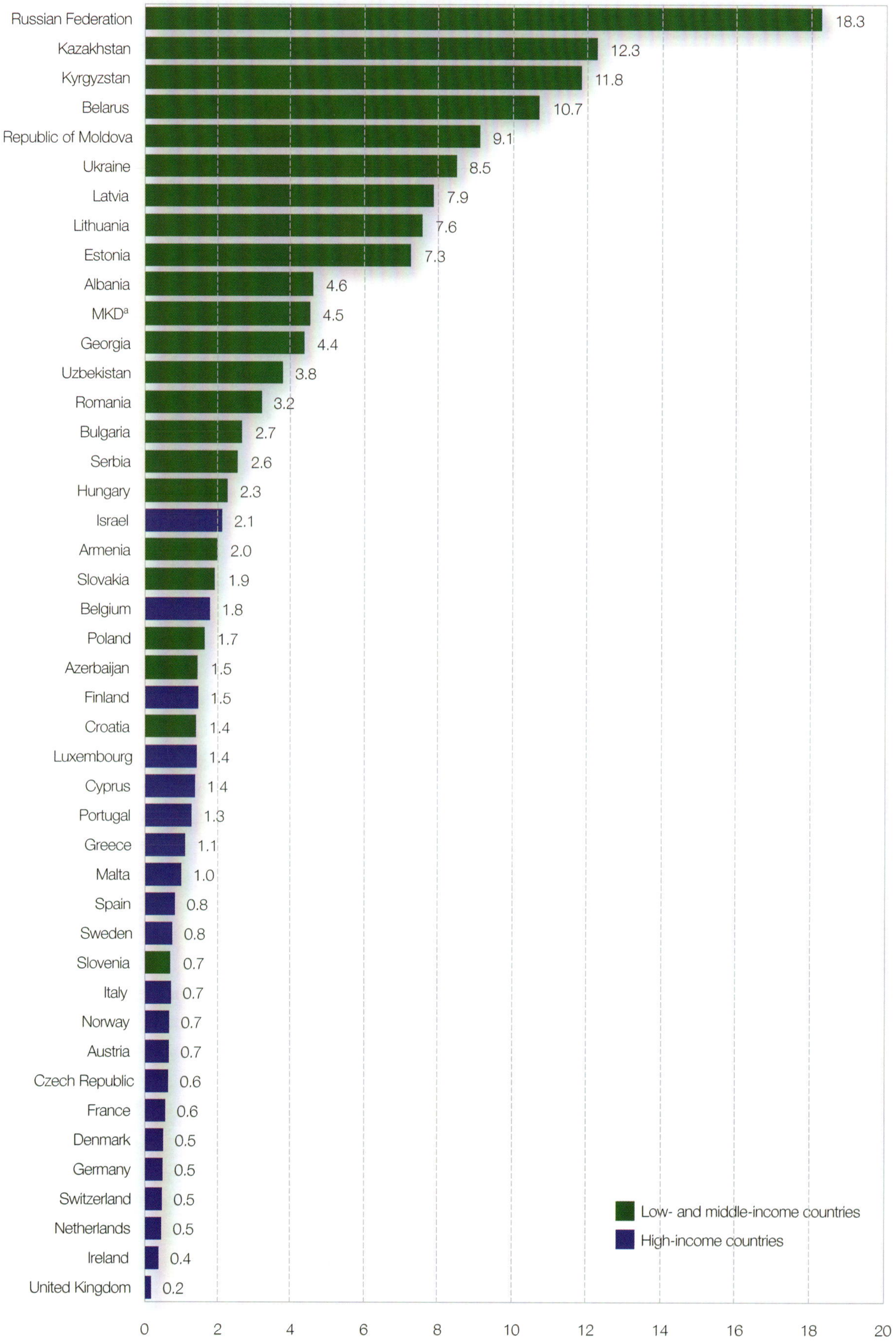

[a] MKD stands for the former Yugoslav Republic of Macedonia; it is an abbreviation of the International Organization for Standardization (ISO), not WHO.

*Source:* European detailed mortality database *(7)*.

**Fig. 2.4. Deaths caused by assault by mode among people aged 60 years and older in 37 countries in the WHO European Region for which data are available**

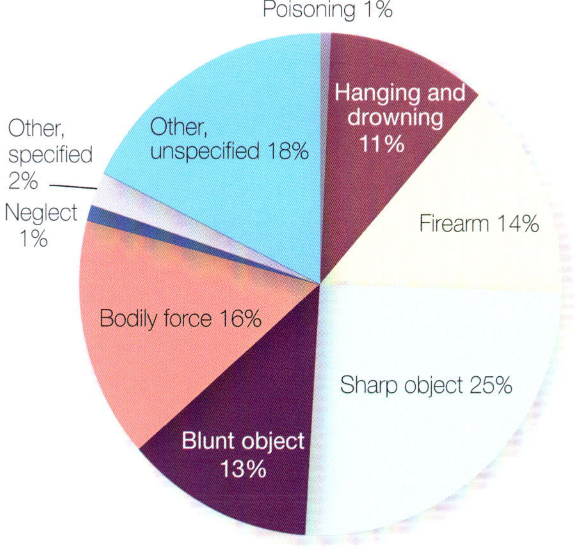


*Source:* European detailed mortality database *(7)*.

### *2.2.5 Interpretation of data on homicides among older people*

Data on homicides caused by elder maltreatment are underreported and incomplete in most countries in the Region. Overall, homicide rates among older people reveal huge inequality in the Region: 12 times higher in low- and middle-income countries. In the absence of better data, it would be reasonable to assume that 30% of all homicides among older people may be attributed to elder maltreatment in all countries throughout the Region (section 2.1). This would suggest that homicides caused by elder maltreatment by a family member are also much higher in low- and middle-income countries. Data also show that the large sex difference in homicide rates among people aged 15–59 years are not so pronounced among older people and the ratio reverses among people aged 80 years and older (Fig. 2.2). The relatively high homicide rates among older women may be caused by elder maltreatment, since intimate partners perpetrate 40–70% of murders among younger women *(10)*. However, older women outlive their partners, and this would contradict this suggestion.

## 2.3 Hospital admissions for assault among older people

Routine information on hospital admissions is only available for a few countries in the WHO European hospital morbidity database *(11)*. Fig. 2.6 shows age-specific hospital admission

**Fig. 2.5. Trends in standardized mortality rates for interpersonal violence among people 65 years and older, WHO European Region**

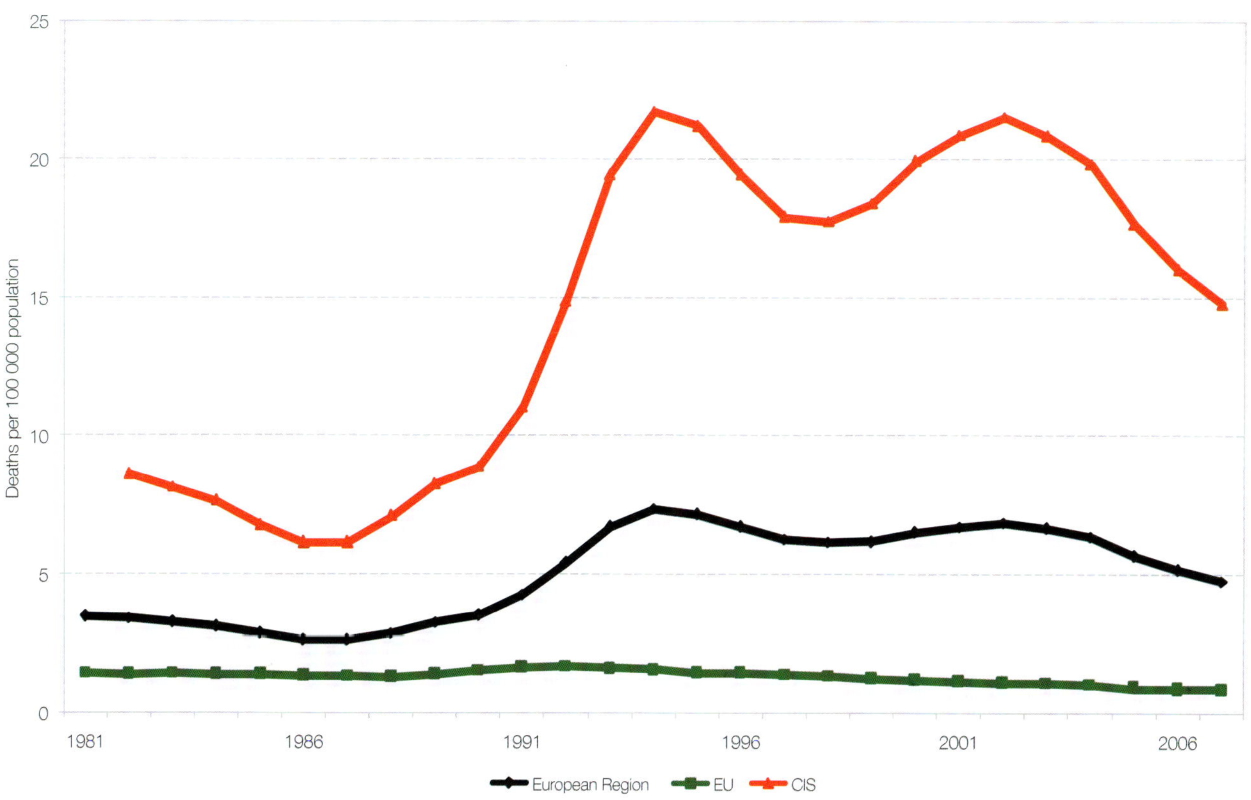


*Source:* Health for All mortality database *(8)*.

**Fig. 2.6. Hospital admission rates for interpersonal violence among people aged 60 years and older in selected countries, WHO European Region, average for 2004–2006 or last three available years**

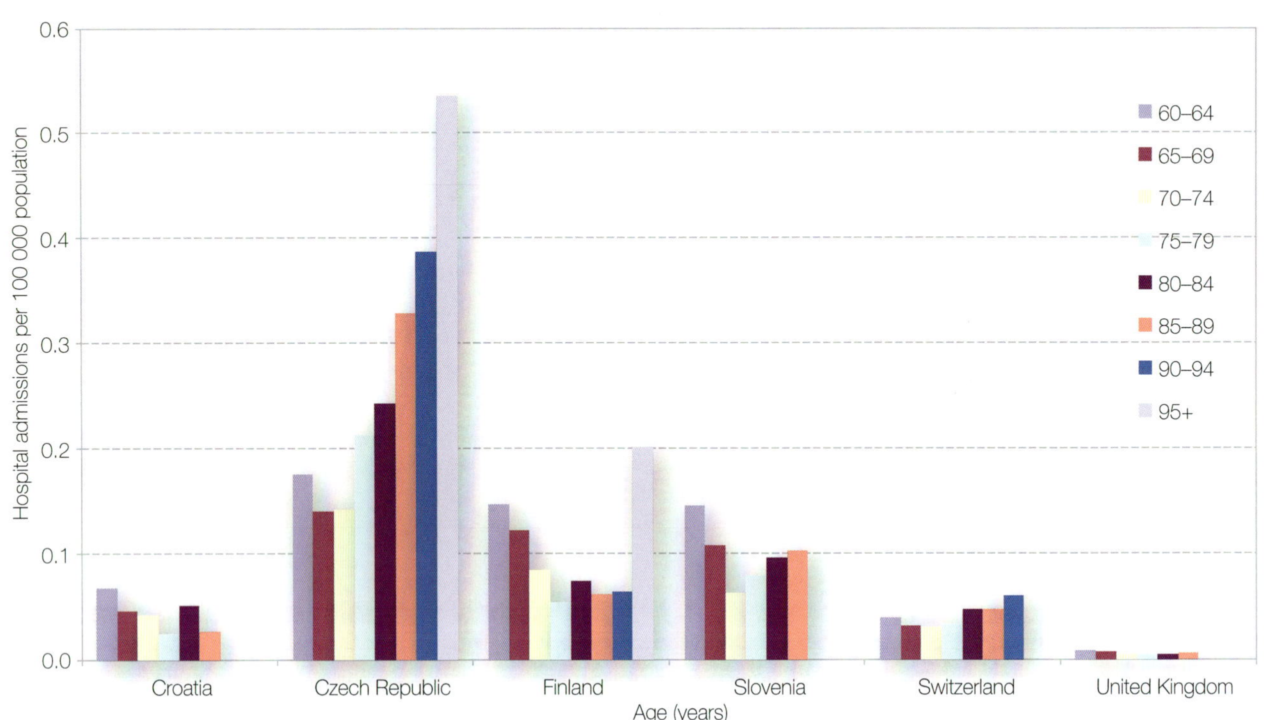


*Source:* European Hospital Morbidity Database *(11)*.

rates from assault. These show that hospital admissions for assault vary by age and also between countries. In most countries, admission rates are high among people 60–64 years old, tend to fall in successive age bands, then rise again and are highest among people aged 90 years and older. The lowest values are reported in the United Kingdom and the highest in the Czech Republic. However, these data are difficult to compare across countries because clinical practice in hospital admission and recording varies.

Data for emergency department attendance for maltreatment and assault are still incomplete. Annex 2 reports information from a few EU countries.

## 2.4 Surveys

As routine information on elder maltreatment is incomplete, the use of community surveys has increased knowledge of the scale of the problem. These make an essential contribution to the public health approach in helping to understand the prevalence of elder maltreatment and associated risk factors. There have been numerous studies with different findings, and these probably reflect different rates of maltreatment in different countries, although some of the difference partly results from different survey methods, demographic characteristics, study settings and criteria used for defining elder maltreatment *(12)*.

### *2.4.1 Surveys in the community*

Pillemer & Finkelhor *(13)* carried out the first methodologically sound study on elder maltreatment in the United States. A total of 2020 interviews were conducted among a large-scale random sample of older people living in Boston metropolitan area who were asked whether they experienced physical violence, verbal aggression and neglect. The overall prevalence of maltreatment of 3.2% was estimated. A subsequent study from the same country using slightly different criteria found an overall prevalence of 10%, and for specific types of maltreatment this was 1.6% for physical abuse, 0.6% for sexual abuse, 5.1% for potential neglect and 5.2% for current financial abuse *(14)*. A study from Korea showed a one-month prevalence of 6.3% of any type of abuse *(15)*.

Table 2.3 summarizes surveys in the community from Europe, but they are briefly discussed here. A study of older people aged over 65 years living in private households (including sheltered and assisted living accommodation) the United Kingdom *(16,17)* reported that 2.6% had experienced mistreatment involving a family member, close friend or care worker during the past year. The prevalence was higher among women than men (3.8% and 1.1% respectively). For the different types of maltreatment, the one-year prevalence was: neglect 1.1%, mental abuse 0.4%, physical abuse

0.4% and sexual abuse 0.2%. A study of older people older than 64 years of age living in private households in Spain *(18)* reported a one-year prevalence of 0.8% by a family member and 1.5% for those more disabled and dependent, confirming the findings of others that the level of maltreatment rises with disability and dependence. The prevalence increased with age: 0.6% among people aged 65–74 years to 1.1% among those older than 74. By type of maltreatment, the prevalence was: 0.2% for physical abuse; 0.3% for mental abuse; 0.2% for financial abuse; 0.1% for sexual abuse and 0.3% for neglect. Unlike the study from the United Kingdom, the proportions of female and male victims were very similar. Women were more likely to be victims of mental, financial and sexual abuse, whereas more men were victims of neglect.

A study from Germany of people 40–85 years old *(19–23)* reported that about one fourth of the survey participants older than 60 years reported verbal aggression by household members within a 12-month period, whereas only 1.3% of older men and 1.6% of older women reported physical violence. Household members committed most violent offences, and this proportion increased with age *(24)*.

The ABUEL (Abuse and health among elderly in Europe) study used a standardized approach in urban populations in seven EU countries: Germany, Greece, Italy, Lithuania, Portugal, Spain and Sweden (Table 2.3) *(25)*. Pooled results reported a one-year prevalence of 19.4% for mental abuse, 2.7% for physical abuse, 0.7% for sexual abuse, 3.8% for financial abuse and 0.7% for injury. The results also show that more men than women were victims of mental abuse (20.0% versus 18.9%); physical abuse (2.8% versus 2.6%); and financial abuse (4.1% versus 3.7%). More women than men were victims of sexual abuse (1.0% versus 0.3%) and injuries (0.9% versus 0.4%). People aged 75–79 and 80–84 years experienced less mental abuse, whereas those aged 80–84 years had a higher rate of financial abuse. Information on perpetrators showed that the perpetrators of mental and physical abuse resulting in injury were mainly the spouse or partner and were mainly friends, acquaintances or neighbours for sexual abuse, while others, children or grandchildren mainly carried out financial abuse (Table 2.3).

A study in the Netherlands *(26)* assessed the one-year prevalence in a sample of older people aged 69–89 years living in Amsterdam. A 5.6% prevalence of elder maltreatment in the previous year was estimated, 3.2% for verbal abuse, 1.2% for physical abuse, 1.4% for financial abuse and 0.2% for neglect. In a semirural community in Finland, the prevalence of elder maltreatment in the previous year was studied after retirement age. This was estimated as 6.7% and was 3.3% among men and 8.8% among women *(27)*. In Israel, a study reported a prevalence of 18.4% of at least one type of maltreatment, ranging from physical and sexual abuse (about 2%) to verbal abuse (about 4%), economic exploitation (about 6%) and neglect (18%) *(28)*. The study reported cultural differences, and older Arab women were the most vulnerable compared with Jews.

Fig. 2.7 summarizes the results of European Region studies reporting physical abuse in the previous year and shows that this ranges from 0.4% to 5.6%. The possible reasons for these differences have been discussed.[7] Table 2.3 provides details on other types of maltreatment.

### *2.4.2 Surveys of family caregivers and others reporting elder maltreatment*

Annex 2 (Table 4) shows the rates of abusive behaviour reported by family caregivers. These generally are much higher than those reported by older people themselves. In a study from Germany, 53% of family caregivers reported at least one incident of maltreatment towards their care-dependent family member during the past 12 months. Verbal aggression or mental abuse (48%) and physical abuse (19%) were reported most often, followed by neglect (6%). There was a higher risk of maltreatment if the relationship with the care recipient was perceived as being negative, with alcohol used to cope with caregiving, assaults by the care recipients or high levels of disability and dependence *(33)*. A study in Spain interviewed family caregivers, and 4.6% reported having abused the older person on some occasion in the previous year; this rose to 5.7% among caregivers looking after highly disabled and dependent older people *(18)*. From the Nordic countries, participants aged 16–74 years in Sweden and Denmark were asked whether they knew about specific cases of older people in their community or among acquaintances who had been battered, threatened, economically exploited, robbed or severely neglected. In both countries, a one-year prevalence of 8% was observed, and these results helped to make elder maltreatment visible in the Nordic countries *(34)*. A systematic review that included several European studies reported that one third of family caregivers of disabled, dependent and/or cognitively impaired older people reported perpetrating significant maltreatment; of this, about 40% was verbal and 11% was physical *(12)*. This shows that this subgroup of older people is vulnerable to maltreatment and that family caregivers are willing to report it. This suggests that asking family caregivers about maltreatment more frequently will probably lead to its detection, with the aim of providing support services for prevention and protection *(12,35)*.

[7] Caution is needed in comparing and interpreting different studies to ensure that they are comparable. This largely depends on several factors such as the population under study (community or institution), the definition of elder maltreatment used or the type of maltreatment studied (physical, sexual, mental and financial or neglect), the questionnaire or instrument used to detect it, the duration over which prevalence is reported (one month, one year or since retirement), the setting where the abuse is occurring (home or institution), the age and sex of the group being studied, the method used to sample the population being studied, geographical area (urban or rural), culture and the level of disability and dependence.

**Table 2.3. Studies asking general population samples of older people about maltreatment**

| Location | Population under study | Maltreatment measure | Prevalence period | Prevalence of maltreatment | Reference |
|---|---|---|---|---|---|
| Across countries | 4467 randomly selected women and men from the general population living in urban centre, aged 60–84 years, no dementia or other cognitive impairment, with a legal status, living in communities or sheltered houses | 52 items based on the United Kingdom study *(16)* and on the revised Conflict Tactics Scales | Once, twice, 3–5, 6–10, 11–20 or more than 20 times during the past year; did not occur during the past year, but before; or never occurred | Mental 19.4%, physical 2.7%, sexual 0.7%, financial 3.8%, injury 0.7% | *(25)* |
| Austria | Community size–stratified random sampling, 593 women older than 60 years living in private households | Standardized questionnaire and telephone interview | One year | Any kind 23.8%, emotional abuse 19.3%, neglect 6.1%, financial abuse 4.7% | *(41)* |
| Finland, semi-rural community | 1022 people older than 65 years | Questionnaire, interviews, clinical scales | After retirement | Total 6.7%: men 3.3%, women 8.8% Physical: men 15%, women 18% Mental: men 46%, women 49% Financial: men 8%, women 9% Neglect: men 0%; women 4% | *(27)* |
| Germany | Random sample of 5711 people 60+ years living in private households | Conflict Tactics Scales | During four years; abusive acts over any one year of that time | Total 3.1%, physical 3.4%, financial 1.3%, neglect 2.7%, verbal 0.8% | *(30)* |
| Germany | Nationwide representative survey of 3030 community-dwelling people 40–85 years old | Conflict Tactics Scales | One year | About 25% of people older than 60 years reported verbal aggression by households members; 1.3% of older men and 1.6% of older women reported physical violence | *(24)* |
| Germany, Bonn | 425 people aged 60+ years | Own questions, postal questionnaire, 10% response rate | Previous five years | About 10% | *(60)* |
| Germany, Stuttgart | 648 randomly selected women and men from the general population living in an urban centre, aged 60–84 years, no dementia or other cognitive impairment, with legal status, living in communities or sheltered houses | 52 items based on the United Kingdom study *(16)* and on the revised Conflict Tactics Scales | Once, twice, 3–5, 6–10, 11–20 or more than 20 times during the past year; did not occur during the past year, but before; or never occurred | Mental 27.1%, physical 3.3%, sexual 0.9%, financial 3.6%, injury 0.4% | *(25)* |
| Greece, Athens | 643 randomly selected women and men from the general population living in an urban centre, aged 60–84 years, no dementia or other cognitive impairment, with legal status, living in communities or sheltered houses | 52 items based on the United Kingdom study *(16)* and on the revised Conflict Tactics Scales | Once, twice, 3–5, 6–10, 11–20 or more than 20 times during the past year; did not occur during the past year, but before; or never occurred | Mental 13.2%, physical 3.4%, sexual 1.5%, financial 4%, injury 1.1% | *(25)* |

**Table 2.3.** *continued*

| Location | Population under study | Maltreatment measure | Prevalence period | Prevalence of maltreatment | Reference |
|---|---|---|---|---|---|
| Ireland | 2000 people 65 years and older were interviewed in their own home | Face-to-face interview, representative sample | One year | Total 2.2%, neglect 0.3%, mental 1.2%, physical 0.5%, sexual 0.05%, financial 1.3% | *(32)* |
| Ireland, Italy, United Kingdom | Opportunistic sample of women (149) older than 59 years from professional and voluntary organizations in Ireland, Italy and the United Kingdom | Own questions | Since turning 59 years | Less than 20% had experienced any form of financial, mental or physical abuse | *(61)* |
| Israel | Representative random urban sample of 1045 Jewish and Arab community-dwelling people aged 65+ years | Revised Conflict Tactics Scales and short situational descriptions and respondents' reactions to them | One year; three months for neglect | 18.4% exposed to at least one type of abuse, excluding neglect; physical and sexual 1.8%, verbal 17.1%, financial 0.5%, neglect 25.6% | *(28)* |
| Italy, Ancona | 628 randomly selected women and men from the general population living in an urban centre, aged 60–84 years, no dementia or other cognitive impairments, with a legal status, living in communities or sheltered houses | 52 items based on the United Kingdom study *(16)* and on the revised Conflict Tactics Scales | Once, twice, 3–5, 6–10, 11–20 or more than 20 times during the past year; did not occur during the past year, but before; or never occurred | Mental 10.4%, physical 1%, sexual 0.5%, financial 2.7%, injury 0% | *(25)* |
| Lithuania, Kaunas | 630 randomly selected women and men from the general population living in an urban centre, aged 60–84 years, no dementia or other cognitive impairment, with legal status, living in communities or sheltered houses | 52 items based on the United Kingdom study *(16)* and on the revised Conflict Tactics Scales | Once, twice, 3–5, 6–10, 11–20 or more than 20 times during the past year; did not occur during the past year, but before; or never occurred | Mental 24.6%, physical 3.8%, sexual 0.3%, financial 2.8%, injury 1.5% | *(25)* |
| Netherlands, Amsterdam | Population-based sample of 1797 people aged 69–89 years, living independently | Conflict Tactics Scales, measure of wife abuse; violence against men; own items | One year | Total 5.6%, verbal 3.2%, physical 1.2%, financial 1.4%, neglect 0.2% | *(29)* |
| Portugal | Random probability sample based on the national post office database: 1586 women older than 60 years living in private households | Standardized questionnaire | One year | Any kind 39.4%, mental 32.9%, financial 16.5%, violation of personal rights 12.8%, neglect 9.9%, sexual 3.6%, physical 2.8% | *(31)* |
| Portugal, Porto | 656 randomly selected women and men from the general population living in an urban centre, aged 60–84 years, no dementia or other cognitive impairment, with a legal status, living in communities or sheltered houses | 52 items based on the United Kingdom study *(16)* and on the revised Conflict Tactics Scales | Once, twice, 3–5, 6–10, 11–20 or more than 20 times during the past year; did not occur during the past year, but before; or never occurred | Mental 21.9%, physical 2.1%, sexual 1.3%, financial 7.8%, injury 0.7% | *(25)* |

**Table 2.3.** *continued*

| Location | Population under study | Maltreatment measure | Prevalence period | Prevalence of maltreatment | Reference |
|---|---|---|---|---|---|
| Spain | 2401 interviews of a general sample of people older than 64 years (private homes) | Face-to-face interview | One year | Total 0.8%, physical 0.2%, mental 0.3%, neglect 0.3%, financial 0.2%, sexual 0.1% | *(18)* |
| Spain, Granada | 636 randomly selected women and men from the general population living in an urban centre, aged 60–84 years, no dementia or other cognitive impairment, with legal status, living in communities or sheltered houses | 52 items based on the United Kingdom study *(16)* and on the revised Conflict Tactics Scales | Once, twice, 3–5, 6–10, 11–20 or more than 20 times during the past year; did not occur during the past year, but before; or never occurred | Mental 11.5%, physical 1.4%, sexual 0.3%, financial 4.8%, injury 0.5% | *(25)* |
| Sweden, Stockholm | 626 randomly selected women and men from the general population living in an urban centre, aged 60–84 years, no dementia or other cognitive impairment, with legal status, living in communities or sheltered houses | 52 items based on the United Kingdom study *(16)* and on the revised Conflict Tactics Scales | Once, twice, 3–5, 6–10, 11–20 or more than 20 times during the past year; did not occur during the past year, but before; or never occurred | Mental 29.7%, physical 4%, sexual 0.5%, financial 1.8%, injury 0.6% | *(25)* |
| United Kingdom | 2111 people older than 66 years in private households; family member, close friend or care worker | Face-to-face interview, representative sample | One year | Total 2.6, neglect 1.1%, mental 0.4%, physical 0.4%, sexual 0.2%, financial 0.7%; if neighbours and acquaintances are considered, the prevalence rises to 4% | *(17)* |

### *2.4.3 Surveys of professional caregivers at home and elsewhere*

Many of the surveys of professional caregivers are from countries outside the European Region. A systematic review showed that about 10% of staff members report physical abuse and 40% mental abuse in the past year *(12)*. Findings from the European Region are not dissimilar. A survey among nurses caring for older people at home in Germany found 40% self-reported involvement in at least one case of maltreatment with their patients in the previous 12 months. Mental abuse or verbal aggression (21%) and neglectful care (19%) were the most common forms encountered, with 8% of the respondents reported encountering at least one case of physical violence and physically coercive behaviour. The nurses thought that problem behaviour could be predicted by patients' aggressive behaviour, the number of people with dementia, the use of alcohol as a means of alleviating work-related stress and nurses' general judgements of the quality of care delivered by in-home service *(23)*.

Another study of a survey of nurses working in residential long-term care in Germany *(36)* found that 71% of nurses reported at least one incident of maltreatment during the past 12 months (Box 2.1). Mental abuse or verbal aggression and neglectful care were most common (both reported by 54%); 23% reported physical abuse. Most reports of physical violence referred to action performed in the course of nursing activities (such as intentionally touching a resident in a rough manner or holding a resident's nose to force him to open his mouth). About 3% indicated they had intentionally pinched, pushed or shoved a resident. Very few nurses reported severe forms of physical maltreatment. Another study of third-party reporting showed that, whereas 80% of nurses had witnessed maltreatment in a care home, only 2% reported it *(37)*. This suggests that greater effort needs to be made to provide supportive structures for professional caregivers in nursing homes.

**Fig. 2.7. Prevalence of physical abuse among older people in selected studies, WHO European Region**

|  |  |
|---|---|
| Spain *(18)* | 0.8% |
| Amsterdam, Netherlands *(29)* | 5.6% |
| Germany *(30)* | 3.1% |
| Stuttgart, Germany *(25)* | 3.3% |
| Athens, Greece *(25)* | 3.4% |
| Ancona, Italy *(25)* | 1.0% |
| Kaunas, Lithuania *(25)* | 3.8% |
| Porto, Portugal *(25)* | 2.1% |
| Granada, Spain *(25)* | 1.4% |
| Stockholm, Sweden *(25)* | 4.0% |
| ABUEL (meta-analysis) *(25)* | 2.7% |
| Portugal *(31)* | 2.8% |
| United Kingdom *(17)* | 0.4% |
| Ireland *(32)* | 2.2% |



*Note:* 95% confidence intervals were calculated using standard methods (see Annex 1 for methods).

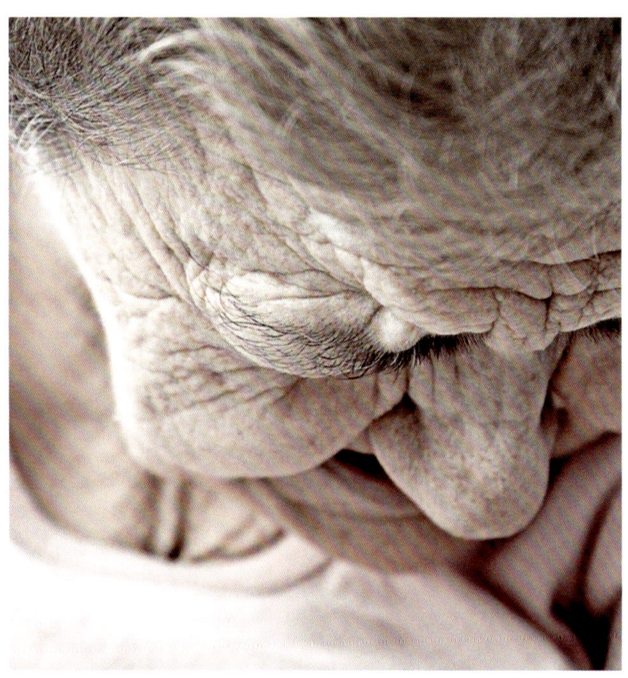

### *2.4.4 Studies examining violence affecting older women*

Studies report that intimate partner violence is prevalent among older people. A study from the United States reported a one-year prevalence of 6% *(38)*. The provisional results from a study in Poland *(39,40)* indicate that 11% had ever experienced maltreatment, the most common type being verbal abuse (9%), and 3% reported physical violence. The Prevalence Study of Violence and Abuse against Older Women (older than 60 years) reports from four countries *(31,41)*. Overall, emotional abuse was the most common form of violence (24%) followed by financial abuse (9%), violation of rights (6%), neglect (5%), sexual abuse (3%) and physical violence (2%). In most cases, the current partner was the perpetrator, especially for physical, emotional and sexual abuse; children or children-in-law were the most frequently mentioned perpetrators in cases of neglect and financial abuse. Box 2.2 reports on violence among older people in the Nordic countries.

**Box 2.1. Case study of criminal justice proceedings from nursing homes in Germany**

A male nursing home director mentions a male head nurse attacking a mentally ill resident: "The [male] resident approached the nurse, and he inadequately tried to keep him at arm's length by kicking him – an excessive reaction. As he was a senior staff member, we had to say 'no, that's intolerable.'"

Beyond these interview and survey data, 35 public prosecutor files on cases of elder maltreatment in nursing homes were analysed *(36)*. Two prototypical cases emerged. The first refers to neglect and insufficient medical treatment with lawsuits filed for bodily injury or negligent homicide by relatives. Victims were described as often being older than 80 years old, suffering from multiple diseases and with severe bedsores. These cases usually ended with a dismissal of criminal proceedings. The second type referred to cases of physical and sexual abuse by nursing home staff or managers. Typically, either the victim or a colleague of the offender reported this to law enforcement agencies. These cases normally resulted in successful conviction. Cases of neglect presented more serious problems for police investigations. The chances are small that criminal proceedings lead to conviction: if the victim dies, has dementia or is otherwise unable to communicate, if there are no competent third-party eyewitnesses, if there is a large delay between the offence and the time it is first reported to police, if indicators of abuse and neglect are insufficient or at best ambiguous, if nursing activities are inadequately documented and if responsibility for an omission is difficult to determine within complex institutional hierarchies.

**Box 2.2. Studies of violence among older people in the Nordic countries**

A Nordic research project on level of living was carried out in 1993 based on comparable official statistics and revealed that many older women feared being exposed to violence in some of the Nordic countries, such as 47% of women 74–85 years old in Sweden. Women in Finland and Iceland reported less fear, although these countries had the highest crime rates amongst their neighbours *(42)*. A literature review of Nordic prevalence studies indicated that 1–9% of older women had been exposed to some form of violence *(43)*.

Statistics from Norway reveal that older people living in Oslo are more exposed to violence and the threat of violence than those living in other parts of the country *(44)*: about 5% of older people in Oslo reported having been exposed to violence. They are, however, not more anxious about violence (27%) than those living in other cities in Norway (29%). The fear of violence appears to become stronger with increasing age of the respondents *(45)*. The empirical evidence suggests that about 4–6% of older people have been exposed to violence or maltreatment annually at 65 years and older *(46)*. Mental health problems and substance abuse among perpetrators might be some of the contextual components. Researchers assume that elder maltreatment is one of the most hidden forms of interpersonal violence and that only a very small number of the incidents are reported to the police and other help services, such as crisis centres, health care providers and social services. One reason for this might be the vulnerable life situations caused by disability and dependence on institutional care or receiving support from family caregivers; another possible reason is the potential shame or guilt connected to the role of being a victim.

### *2.4.5 Estimates for the types of elder maltreatment in the European Region*

The prevalence of subtypes of elder maltreatment in the WHO European Region was roughly estimated, applying the best available estimates of prevalence to the Region's population. These estimates are derived from a study of seven EU countries *(25)* for which the prevalence was found by type of maltreatment: physical 2.7%, sexual 0.7%, mental 19.4% and financial 3.8%. These suggest that, in the WHO European Region in any given year, at least 4 million people aged 60 years and older experience elder maltreatment in the form of physical abuse, 1 million sexual abuse, 6 million financial abuse and 29 million mental abuse. Despite the limitations of such extrapolations, this suggests that elder maltreatment is a grave concern.[8]

[8] Annex 1 discusses the limitations of this approach. This multi-country survey was conducted in urban areas, and there are limitations in extrapolating to other countries, settings and cultures.

## 2.5 Consequences of elder maltreatment

The consequences of elder maltreatment can be serious and have far-reaching effects for older people *(1,14,35,47)*. Compared with younger adults, older people are physically weaker, and even a minor injury could therefore have grave consequences and result in longer convalescence. The immediate physical effects include assault injuries ranging from bruises to broken bones and head injuries, persistent physical pain and soreness, poor nutrition and dehydration, sleep disturbances and susceptibility to new illnesses *(2,48–50)*. Elder maltreatment has been implicated in premature mortality, which may not only be caused by frailty but also comorbid conditions that may be further aggravated *(51)*. In a study from the United States, violent assaults accounted for 14% of trauma patients older than 64 years, and these injuries were reported to more likely result in death than among younger people *(48)*.

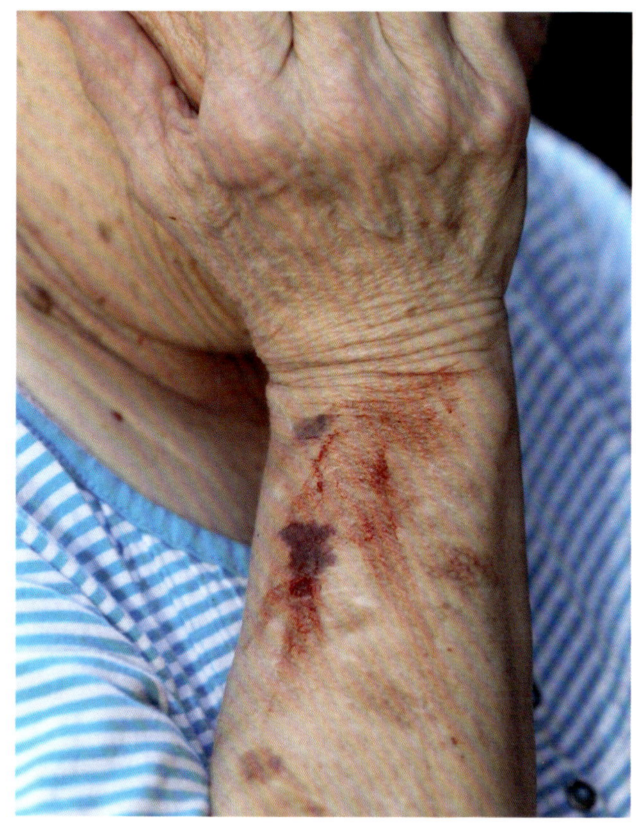

The mental effects may also be grave, with increased experiences of fear and grief *(29)*, anger and upset and isolation from family and friends *(16)*. The spectrum includes worsened quality of life, distress and depression, increased risks of developing fear and anxiety reactions, helplessness, sleep disturbance and post-traumatic stress *(52)*. Elder maltreatment may result in great emotional distress and the loss of self-confidence and self-esteem *(29)*. Longer-term and more severe maltreatment may result in worse mental effects, such as depression and thoughts of suicide or self-harm *(52)*. A key theme emerging in the literature is the lasting effects of maltreatment on older people. Some older people who have been maltreated described their experiences as "devastating", with many feeling they would never fully recover *(53)*. Financial abuse and the loss of even small amounts of money could seriously affect older people who survive on limited incomes. Nevertheless, few studies have properly examined these effects, and greater emphasis is needed on longitudinal studies to better understand the diverse effects of the different types of maltreatment and how to distinguish some health effects from the ageing process *(48)*.

## 2.6 Costs to society

Similar to other forms of violence, the costs of elder maltreatment are likely to be profound. Few studies have been undertaken to quantify this *(1,54,55)*. These need to consider the direct costs arising directly from the maltreatment and would include increased health care costs to treat the people who have been maltreated and services to identify and rehabilitate elder maltreatment victims and perpetrators. In care settings, costs would include services for preventing maltreatment (case detection, staff training and adequate staffing) and identifying maltreatment and intervening (developing protocols, investigating and staffing). Older people who have been maltreated may need community services such as home support, case management and long-term care. The criminal justice system and social care system would incur non–health care costs to provide protection and care. There would be costs to compensate for assets lost through exploitation and the financial loss by older people because of misappropriation of resources, as in financial abuse *(56)*. Elder maltreatment also results in indirect costs because of lost resources and opportunities such as reduced productivity of caregivers, loss of health-related quality of life and lost investment in social capital. This may vary from increased social isolation and reduced social resources by withdrawal from and reduced access to social support networks. In extreme cases, there are also costs associated with the loss of life.

### Key messages

Surveillance using routine information sources is unreliable and needs to be improved using standardized definitions in all countries in the European Region.

The prevalence of elder maltreatment in the community and in other settings is high and varies according to culture and country.

More standardized definitions, instruments and methods are needed in European Region surveys.

Vulnerable older people and family caregivers are willing to report elder maltreatment, and more should be done to ask about it.

Professional caregivers report committing acts of abuse, and the scale of this needs to be better understood to provide remedial action.

Elder maltreatment may lead to lasting harmful physical and mental effects among older people.

The societal costs of elder maltreatment need to be better studied in the European Region.

Although the costs of financial maltreatment have not been properly quantified in the European Region, these probably comprise billions of euros annually. Estimates of such costs are not currently available globally. A study from Queensland, Australia *(57)* suggests that elder maltreatment is associated with very great suffering and financial costs. The Elder Abuse Prevention Unit estimated the financial exploitation of older people in Queensland for the 2007/2008 fiscal year to be a minimum of A$ 1.8 billion and a maximum of A$ 5.8 billion. In addition, costs due to hospital admissions for elder maltreatment for 2007/2008 have been estimated to be between A$ 9.9 million and A$ 30.7 million. Cost approximations from the United States suggest that the direct health care costs of injuries caused by elder maltreatment are likely to contribute more than US$ 5.3 billion to the country's annual health care expenditure *(58,59)*. These figures do not include indirect costs, and no estimates are available for these worldwide for elder maltreatment.

## 2.7 References


1. Krug E et al., eds. *World report on violence and health*. Geneva, World Health Organization, 2002 (http://www.who.int/violence_injury_prevention/violence/world_report/en, accessed 9 May 2011).

2. Ahmad M, Lachs MS. Elder abuse and neglect: what physicians can and should do. *Cleveland Clinic Journal of Medicine*, 2002, 69:801–808.

3. Iborra I, ed. *Violencia contra personas mayores [Violence against older people]*. Barcelona, Editorial Ariel, 2005 (Colección Estudios sobre Violencia, No. 11).

4. Collins KA, Presnell SE. Elder homicide. A 20-year study. *American Journal of Forensic Medicine and Pathology*, 2006, 27:183–187.

5. Falzon AL, Davis GG. A 15 year retrospective review of homicide in the elderly. *Journal of Forensic Sciences*, 1998, 43:371–374.

6. *The global burden of disease: 2004 update*. Geneva, World Health Organization, 2008 (http://www.who.int/healthinfo/global_burden_disease/2004_report_update/en/index.html, accessed 9 May 2011).

7. European detailed mortality database [online database]. Copenhagen, WHO Regional Office for Europe, 2010 (http://www.euro.who.int/hfadb, accessed 9 May 2011).

8. Mortality indicator database [online database]. Copenhagen, WHO Regional Office for Europe, 2010 (http://www.euro.who.int/hfadb, accessed 9 May 2011).

9. McKee M et al. Health policy-making in central and eastern Europe: why has there been so little action on injuries? *Health Policy and Planning*, 2000, 15:263–269.

10. Sethi D et al. *Injuries and violence in Europe: why they matter and what can be done*. Copenhagen, WHO Regional Office for Europe, 2006 (http://www.euro.who.int/__data/assets/pdf_file/0007/98404/E87321.pdf, accessed 9 May 2011).

11. European hospital morbidity database [online database]. Copenhagen, WHO Regional Office for Europe, 2010 (http://www.euro.who.int/hfadb, accessed 9 May 2011).

12. Cooper C, Selwood A, Livingston G. The prevalence of elder abuse and neglect: a systematic review. *Age and Aging*, 2008, 37:151–160.

13. Pillimer K, Finkelhor D. The prevalence of elder abuse: a random sample survey. *The Gerontologist*, 1988, 28:51–57.

14. Acierno R et al. Prevalence and correlates of emotional, physical, sexual, and financial abuse and potential neglect in the United States: the National Elder Mistreatment Study. *American Journal of Public Health*, 2010, 100:292–297.

15. Oh J et al. A study of elder abuse in Korea. *International Journal of Nursing Studies*, 2006, 43:203–214.

16. O'Keeffe M et al. *UK Study of Abuse and Neglect of Older People: prevalence survey report*. London, National Centre for Social Research and King's College London, 2007.

17. Biggs S et al. Mistreatment of the older people in the United Kingdom: findings from the first National Prevalence Study. *Journal of Elder Abuse and Neglect*, 2009, 21:1–14.

18. Iborra I. *Maltrato de personas mayores en la familia en España [Elder maltreatment within families in Spain]*. Valencia, Queen Sofía Center, 2008 (Serie Documentos No. 13).

19. Görgen T, ed. *Sicherer Hafen oder gefahrvolle Zone? Kriminalitäts- und Gewalterfahrungen im Leben alter Menschen [Safe haven or danger zone? Experiences of crime and violence in older peoples' lives]*. Frankfurt am Main, Verlag für Polizeiwissenschaft, 2010.

20. Görgen T. Viktimisierung von Senioren – empirische Daten und Schlussfolgerungen für eine alternde Gesellschaft [Victimization of older people – empirical data and implications for an ageing society]. In: Frevel B, Bredthauer R, eds. *Empirische Polizeiforschung XII: Demografischer Wandel und Polizei [Empirical police research XII: demographic changes and the police]*. Frankfurt am Main, Verlag für Polizeiwissenschaft, 2010:123–147.

21. Görgen T, Herbst S, Rabold S. *Kriminalitäts- und Gewaltgefährdungen im höheren Lebensalter und in der häuslichen Pflege [Risks of crime and violence in old age and in domestic care]*. Hanover, Criminological Research Institute of Lower Saxony, 2006 (KFN Research Report, No. 98).

22. Görgen T, Rabold S, Herbst S. *Viktimisierungen im Alter und in der häuslichen Pflege: Wege in ein schwieriges Forschungsfeld [Victimization in old age and in domestic care: pathways into a difficult research area]*. Hanover, Criminological Research Institute of Lower Saxony, 2006 (KFN Research Report, No. 99).

23. Rabold S, Görgen T. Misshandlung und Vernachlässigung älterer Menschen durch ambulante Pflegekräfte: Ergebnisse einer Befragung von Mitarbeiterinnen und Mitarbeitern ambulanter Dienste [Abuse and neglect of older people by home care staff: results of a survey among nurses in home care services]. *Zeitschrift für Gerontologie und Geriatrie*, 2007, 40:366–374.

24. Görgen T, Herbst S, Rabold S. Jenseits der Kriminalstatistik: Befunde einer bundesweiten Opferwerdungsbefragung [Beyond crime statistics: results of a nationwide victimization survey]. In: Görgen T, ed. *Sicherer Hafen oder gefahrvolle Zone? Kriminalitäts- und Gewalterfahrungen im Leben alter Menschen [Safe haven or danger zone? Experiences of crime and violence in older peoples' lives]*. Frankfurt am Main, Verlag für Polizeiwissenschaft, 2010:122–174.

25. Soares JJF et al. *Abuse and health in Europe*. Kaunas, Lithuanian University of Health Sciences Press, 2010.

26. Comijs HC et al. Elder abuse in the community: prevalence and consequences. *Journal of the American Geriatrics Society*, 1998, 46:885–888.

27. Kivela SL et al. Abuse in old age – epidemiological data from Finland. *Journal of Elder Abuse and Neglect*, 1992, 4:1–18.

28. Lowenstein A et al. Is elder abuse and neglect a social phenomenon? Data from the first national prevalence survey in Israel. *Journal of Elder Abuse and Neglect*, 2009, 21:253–277.

29. Comijs HC et al. Psychological distress in victims of elder mistreatment: the effects of social support and coping. *Journal of Gerontology Series B Psychological Sciences and Social Sciences*, 1999, 54:240–245.

30. Wetzels P, Greve W. [Older people as victims of family violence: – results of a criminological dark field study.] *Zeitschrift für Gerontologie and Geriatrie*, 1996, 29:191–200.

31. Ferreira-Alves J, Santos AJ. *Prevalence study of abuse and violence against older women: results of the Portugal survey (AVOW Project)*. Braga, Minho University, 2010.

32. Naughton C et al. *Abuse and neglect of older people in Ireland. Report on the National Study of Elder Abuse and Neglect*. Dublin, National Centre for the Protection of Older People, 2010.

33. Görgen T, Bauer R, Schröder M. Wenn Pflege in der Familie zum Risiko wird: Befunde einer schriftlichen Befragung pflegender Angehöriger [When family caregiving becomes risky: results of a questionnaire study among family caregivers]. In: Görgen T, ed. *Sicherer Hafen oder gefahrvolle Zone? Kriminalitäts- und Gewalterfahrungen im Leben alter Menschen [Safe haven or danger zone? Experiences of crime and violence in older peoples' lives]*. Frankfurt am Main, Verlag für Polizeiwissenschaft, 2010:196–207.

34. Tornstram L. Abuse of the elderly in Denmark and Sweden: results from a population study. *Journal of Elder Abuse and Neglect*, 1989, 1:35–44.

35. Lachs MS, Pillemer K. Current concepts – abuse and neglect of elderly persons. *New England Journal of Medicine*, 1995, 332:437–443.

36. Görgen T. "As if I just didn't exist" – elder abuse and neglect in nursing homes. In: Wahidin A, Cain M, eds. *Ageing, crime and society*. Cullompton, Willan, 2006:71–89.

37. Goergen T. Stress, conflict, elder abuse and neglect in German nursing homes: a pilot study among professional caregivers. *Journal of Elder Abuse and Neglect*, 2001, 13:1–26.

38. Harris S. For better or worse: spouse abuse grown old. *Journal of Elder Abuse and Neglect*, 1996, 8:1–33.

39. Halicka M, Halicki J, Kramkowska E. *National report – Poland. IPVoW intimate partner violence against older women*. Bialystok, University of Bialystok, 2010.

40. Intimate Partner Violence against older Women [web site]. Münster, German Police University, 2011 (http://www.ipvow.org, accessed 9 May 2011).

41. Lang G, Enzenhofer E. *Prevalence study of abuse and violence against older women: results of the Austrian survey (AVOW Project)*. Vienna, Research Institute of the Red Cross, 2011.

42. Helset A. Elderly women in the Nordic countries: level of living and situation in life. *Scandinavian Journal of Social Medicine*, 1993, 21:223–226.

43. Luoma M-L, Koivusilta M. *Prevalence study of abuse and violence against old women. Literature review: Finland and the Nordic countries*. Helsinki, National Institute for Health and Welfare, Finland, 2009.

44. *Report No. 25 (2005–2006) to the Storting. Long term care – future challenges. Care Plan 2015*. Oslo, Ministry of Health and Care Services, 2006.

45. *Living Conditions Survey (Levekårsundersøkelsen) 1997*. Kongsvinger, Statistics Norway, 1997.

46. Juklestad ON, Johns S. *Vern for elder. Tiltak mot overgrep i hjemmet [Protecting older people. Measures against maltreatment in the home]*. Oslo, Kommuneforlaget, 1997.

47. Bonnie R, Wallace R, eds. *Elder mistreatment: abuse, neglect, and exploitation in an aging America*. Washington, DC, National Academies Press, 2003.

48. Collins KA. Elder maltreatment. A review. *Archives of Pathology and Laboratory Medicine*, 2006, 130:1290–1296.

49. *Understanding elder maltreatment. Fact sheet 2010*. Atlanta, United States Centers for Disease Control and Prevention, 2010 (http://www.cdc.gov/violenceprevention/pdf/em-factsheet-a.pdf, accessed 9 May 2011).

50. Samaras N et al. Older patients in the emergency department: a review. *Annals of Emergency Medicine*, 2010, 56:261–269.

51. Lachs MS et al. The mortality of elder mistreatment. *Journal of the American Medical Association*, 1998, 280:428–432.

52. Mowlam A et al. *UK Study of Abuse and Neglect of Older People: qualitative findings*. London, National Centre for Social Research and King's College London, 2007.

53. Mears J. Survival is not enough: violence against older women in Australia. *Violence against Women*, 2003, 9:1478–1489.

54. Waters H et al. *The economic dimensions of interpersonal violence*. Geneva, World Health Organization, 2004 (http://www.who.int/violence_injury_prevention/publications/violence/economic_dimensions/en, accessed 9 May 2011).

55. American Medical Association white paper on elderly health. Report of the Council on Scientific Affairs. *Archives of Internal Medicine*, 1990, 150:2459–2472.

56. Butchart A et al. *Manual for estimating the economic costs of injuries due to interpersonal and self-directed violence*. Geneva, World Health Organization, 2008 (http://www.who.int/violence_injury_prevention/violence/activities/economics/en/inden.html, accessed 9 May 2011).

57. Jackson L. *The cost of elder abuse in Queensland: who pays and how much*. Brisbane, Elder Abuse Prevention Unit, 2009.

58. Dong XQ et al. Report of elder self-neglect and mortality in a community-dwelling population. *Journal of investigative Medicine*, 2009, 57:558–559.

59. Mouton CP et al. Prevalence and 3-year incidence of abuse among postmenopausal women. *American Journal of Public Health*, 2004, 94:605–612.

# 3. Risk factors

## 3.1 Introduction

Understanding which factors are related to elder maltreatment is an essential step in the public health approach to preventing it *(1)*. No single factor explains why some individuals behave violently toward others or why elder maltreatment is more prevalent in some communities than in others *(1)*. Elder maltreatment is the result of the complex interaction of individual, relationship, social, cultural and environmental factors. This chapter presents the current evidence on the main risk factors using an ecological model (see Fig. 1.1, section 1.6). Previous research on the risk factors of elder maltreatment has limitations. These need to be borne in mind and arise from unclear definitions of maltreatment and its types, the population at risk, such as age, setting or disability, and inadequate study designs *(2)*. Despite these, the literature has consistently found some risk factors of importance, and these will be highlighted (Table 3.1). The findings presented emphasize the European literature and are categorized as strong, potential and contested.[9]

**Key facts**

The evidence base for risk factors needs to be better developed.

At the individual level, strong evidence indicates that dementia is a risk factor for becoming a victim of elder maltreatment.

For perpetrators, strong evidence supports the following as risk factors: mental health problems, especially depression; previous violent behaviour; and substance misuse, especially alcohol abuse.

At the relationship level, risk factors supported by strong evidence include the dependence of the perpetrator on the victim and living in shared accommodation.

The key risk factor at the community level supported by strong evidence is social isolation.

At the societal level, ageism, inequality and attitudes towards violence are suggested to have a possible role but need to be better understood.

The risk factors for elder maltreatment occurring in institutions need to be studied.

Protective factors such as positive life experiences and community connectedness should be promoted.

## 3.2 Individual-level risk factors for victimization

The personal and individual-level factors considered to have more influence on a person becoming either a victim or perpetrator of violence against older people are as follows.

### *3.2.1 Gender and victimization*

Some studies indicate that more victims are women as opposed to men *(3–5)*. Research into crimes of maltreatment against older people within the family carried out in 10 countries *(6)* revealed that women comprise 60–75% of victims. In Spain, 63% of victims were women, and the prevalence was higher for women (0.9%) than for men (0.7%) *(7)*. A prevalence study from the United Kingdom *(8)* reported that women were more likely to report maltreatment than men (3.8% of women versus 1.1% of older men). In a prevalence study conducted in Ireland, women (2.4%) were more likely than men (1.9%) to report experiences of maltreatment in the previous 12 months, especially financial and interpersonal types of maltreatment *(9)*.[10] In contrast, the ABUEL study *(10)* reported that more men than women were victims of mental, physical and financial abuse. In this study, more women than men were reported to be victims of sexual abuse and physical injuries. Women seem to experience most of the more severe cases of physical and emotional abuse *(11)*. In cases of homicide by family members, a woman was more likely to be killed by her male partner and older men at the hands of their children *(12)*. In care homes, more maltreatment has been described among women than among men (Box 3.1) *(13)*. Most of these studies have reported different prevalence rates, and further research is indicated that adjusts for other risk factors for the different types of maltreatment.

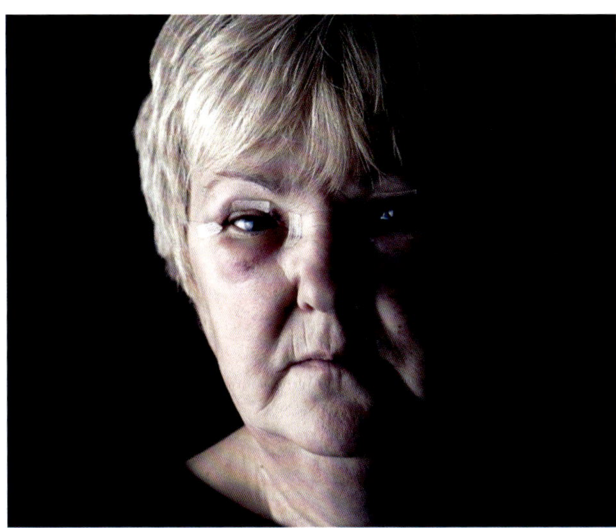

[9] Strong: risk factors validated by substantial evidence that have either unanimous or nearly unanimous support from several studies, including early studies that used case-control methods.
Potential: risk factors for which the available evidence is either mixed or somewhat limited.
Contested: risk factors for which there has been a hypothesis concerning increased risk but for which clear evidence available from the research is lacking.

[10] The findings in the prevalence studies in Ireland and the United Kingdom were statistically significant. For details, see the relevant reports.

**Table 3.1. Risk factors for elder maltreatment**

| Level | Main risk factors |
|---|---|
| Individual (victim) | Sex: women<br>Age: older than 74 years<br>Dependence: high levels of physical or intellectual disability<br>Dementia, including Alzheimer's disease and other types of dementia<br>Mental disorders: depression<br>Aggression and challenging behaviour by the victim |
| Individual (perpetrator) | Sex: men in cases of physical abuse and women in neglect cases<br>Mental disorders: depression<br>Substance abuse: alcohol and drug misuse<br>Hostility and aggression<br>Financial problems<br>Stress: caregiver burnout |
| Relationship | Financial dependence of the perpetrator on the victim<br>Dependence of the perpetrator on the victim (emotional and accommodation)<br>Intergenerational transmission of violence<br>Long-term history of difficulty in the relationship<br>Kinship: children or partner<br>Living arrangement |
| Community | Social isolation: victim lives alone with perpetrator and both have few social contacts<br>Lack of social support: absence of social support resources and systems |
| Societal | Discrimination because of age: ageism<br>Other forms of discrimination: sexism and racism<br>Social and economic factors<br>Violent culture: normalization of violence |

**Box 3.1. Individual-level risk factors for victims who live in care settings**

Being a woman.

Having some type of physical or mental disability or cognitive impairment.

Aggressive or challenging behaviour (perhaps as a result of illness or a health condition).

Rejection of a passive, acquiescent role.

Lack of family members and having few visitors to act as a buffer for risk situations.

*Sources*: Juklestad *(13)* and Rubio *(14)*.

### *3.2.2 Age of victims*

The risk of maltreatment appears to increase with age. In a study in Spain, the prevalence of maltreatment increased from 0.6% among people 65–74 years old, reaching 1.1% for those older than 74 years *(7)*. It appears to rise further from 75 years upwards *(7,15,16)*. The prevalence of maltreatment in Ireland among people older than 70 years was twice that among people aged 65–69 years *(9)*. This also applies to the various types of maltreatment. In Israel, the prevalence of physical abuse appeared to be higher among the oldest women *(17,18)*. For mental abuse, the ABUEL study *(10)* found that people 75–84 years old had lower risk than those aged 65–74 years. In the United Kingdom *(8)*, neglect was more prevalent among women older than 85 years. The risk of financial abuse also appears to increase with age *(19)*, and evidence suggests that this is higher among men older than 80 years *(10)*.

### *3.2.3 Victim's dependence or disability*

Maltreatment rates increase with dependence and disability *(7,20–24)*. In Spain *(7)*, the rate of maltreatment quadrupled among older people with higher levels of dependence[11]

[11] Older people with high levels of dependence are considered those who need help throughout the day to perform the activities of daily living.

(2.9%) compared with older people who were not so dependent (0.7%). This association was also found for homicide, in which older victims of homicide committed by family members had some form of disability *(12)*. In addition, a study of the prevalence of and risk factors for elder maltreatment by caregivers in Chinese families in the Hong Kong Special Administrative Region of China showed that, overall, verbal and physical abuse were best predicted by participants' dependence on the caregivers *(25)*. Further, the association of increased dependence and maltreatment also applies to care homes *(14)*. Increased maltreatment has been reported to be associated with declining health in Ireland *(9)* and to depression in the United Kingdom *(8)*. Financial abuse and interpersonal abuse increased among both men and women who had a long-term illness *(9)*. Worsening health and dependence on someone to carry out activities of daily living have been reported as risk factors for suspected maltreatment *(26,27)*.

In relation to disability, such factors as changes in expectation on the part of caregivers, further reduction in functional capacity with time and ignorance of the effects of an illness on cognition have been proposed to increase the risk of certain types of maltreatment *(28)*. Many of these studies lack a control group, suggesting that more rigorous research is needed.

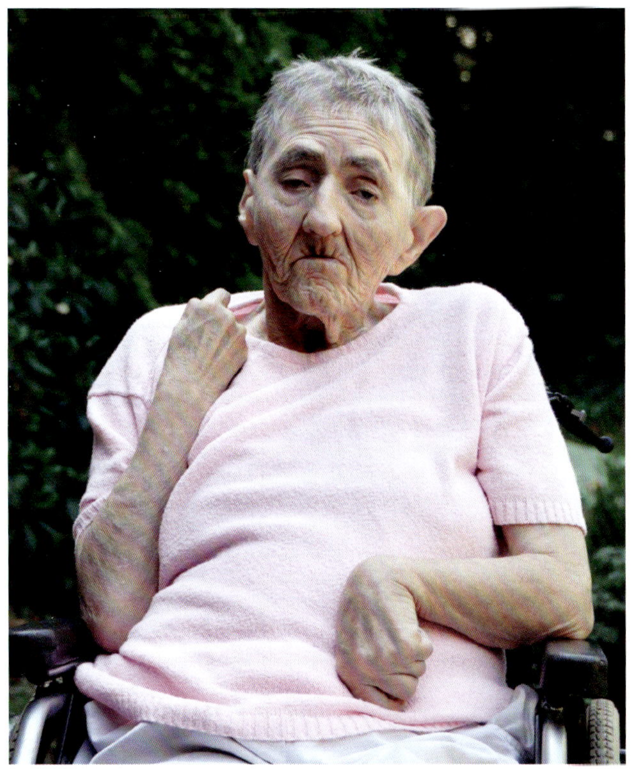

### 3.2.4 Cognitive state of the victims: dementia

Older people with cognitive impairment such as Alzheimer's disease and other forms of dementia have been described as experiencing a higher prevalence of maltreatment (14%) than the general population *(29)*. Similarly, family caregivers of people with dementia report higher levels of perpetration (12%) than the caregivers of relatives without dementia (4%) *(7)*. Further, the likelihood of being murdered by a family member was three times higher if the older person had Alzheimer's disease or other dementia than if they did not. Maltreatment of older people with Alzheimer's disease by their caregivers is thought to be linked to violent, disruptive and challenging behaviour of the older person, which might precipitate a retaliatory response *(30–32)*. A study of nursing home staff in Germany found that self-reported maltreatment by nursing staff was associated with aggressive behaviour by older people and a high workload of older people with dementia *(27)*. The National Center on Elder Abuse study *(16)* undertaken in the United States also found that worsening cognitive ability was a relevant factor.

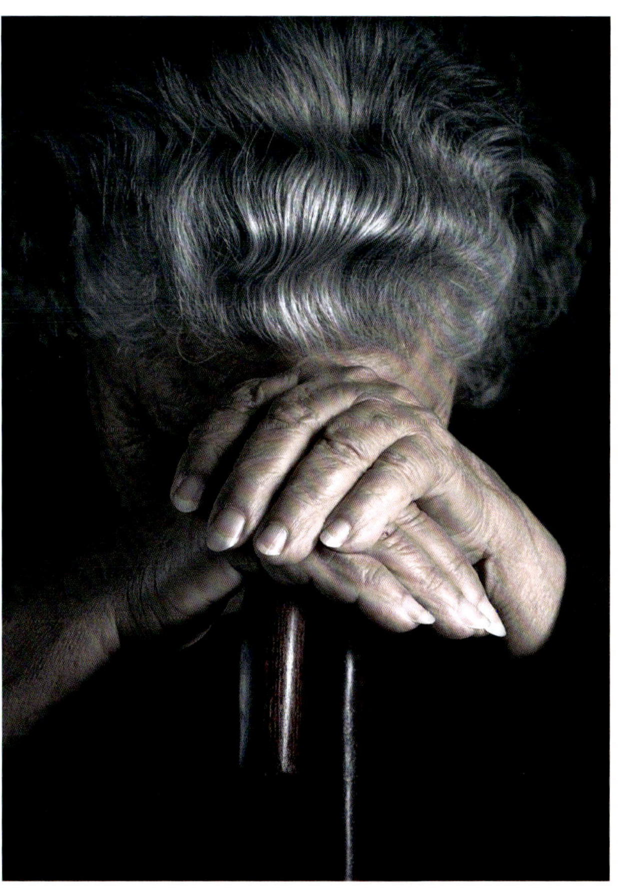

### 3.2.5 Aggression among victims

A study of risk factors for elder maltreatment in community settings showed that the higher the frequency of provocative and aggressive behaviour by an older person, the higher the risk of their caregiver engaging in maltreatment *(33–35)*. Care and nursing staff reported high levels of aggressive behaviour by residents and frequent assaults by care recipients as potential triggers for abusive situations *(27)*. Such factors as stress, the quality of the relationship between the older person and the caregiver and the existing problems such as substance misuse or a mental disorder in the caregiver (mainly depression) influence the likelihood of maltreatment as a response to aggression on the part of the older person *(36)*. The complex interaction of factors limits the available evidence on this risk factor, which warrants further study.

### *3.2.6 Mental health and victims*

Various studies have found that victims of elder maltreatment frequently have anxiety symptoms, depression, suicidal thoughts and feelings of unhappiness, shame or guilt and social isolation *(2,37)*. This may vary with the type of maltreatment. For example, depressive symptoms were associated only in the case of mental abuse *(19)*. In the ABUEL study *(10)*, depressive symptoms were associated with mental abuse and injuries. These symptoms such as depression, suicidal ideation and unhappiness may well be outcomes resulting from maltreatment rather than predisposing risk factors. Better research is needed to elucidate this further.

### *3.2.7 Key risk factors for victims at the individual level*

Dementia in the victim is the risk factor at the individual level that is supported by strong evidence.

## 3.3 Individual-level risk factors for perpetration

### *3.3.1 Gender and perpetration*

Perpetrators have been reported to be more likely to be men than women *(7,38)*, especially for sexual abuse, severe physical abuse and homicide *(12,37,38)*. This was found in Spain in relation to caregivers who perpetrate maltreatment, who were more likely to be men (6%) rather than women (4%) *(7)*. The United Kingdom prevalence study *(39)* indicated that 80% of the perpetrators of interpersonal abuse (physical, mental and sexual abuse combined) were men and 20% were women. The split for financial abuse was more equal (56% men, 44% women). However a study from Ireland reported that men were only slightly more likely to be perpetrators than women *(9)*. Women, however, are more likely to be involved in neglect, and men are more likely to be responsible for severe physical abuse and sexual abuse.

### *3.3.2 Age and perpetration*

In the United Kingdom *(8)*, the age profile of perpetrators indicated that perpetrators of financial abuse were younger than those involved in other types of abuse.

### *3.3.3 Stress among perpetrators*

Caring for an older relative may be an important cause of stress for families, especially if support is lacking. This is more likely if more assistance is needed because of the level of impairment and disability and the consequent physical or mental dependence. Factors that may cause this are scarce information on the effects of ageing and illnesses in later life, lack of caregiver skills or training to assist caregivers and inadequate resources to support caregivers and care recipients. An important factor in precipitating elder maltreatment is the perceived level of care burden and higher stress levels resulting from problem behaviour by the older person *(33,34)*. For example, in Spain, a study *(7)* reported that 72% of caregivers who mistreated the older person in their charge had felt overburdened by the situation. It is reported that professional caregivers affected by "caregiver burden syndrome" may suffer physical and mental health effects *(40)*. Some empirical evidence indicates that the perception of stress and burnout syndrome predict the presence of elder maltreatment *(41)*. This has been previously linked to the dependence of the older person, but it may instead simply result from the caregiver's internal resources and possible previous mental problems *(42)*. Increasing evidence indicates that the most important factor may be the type of relationship between the caregiver and the older person (see section 3.4.5).

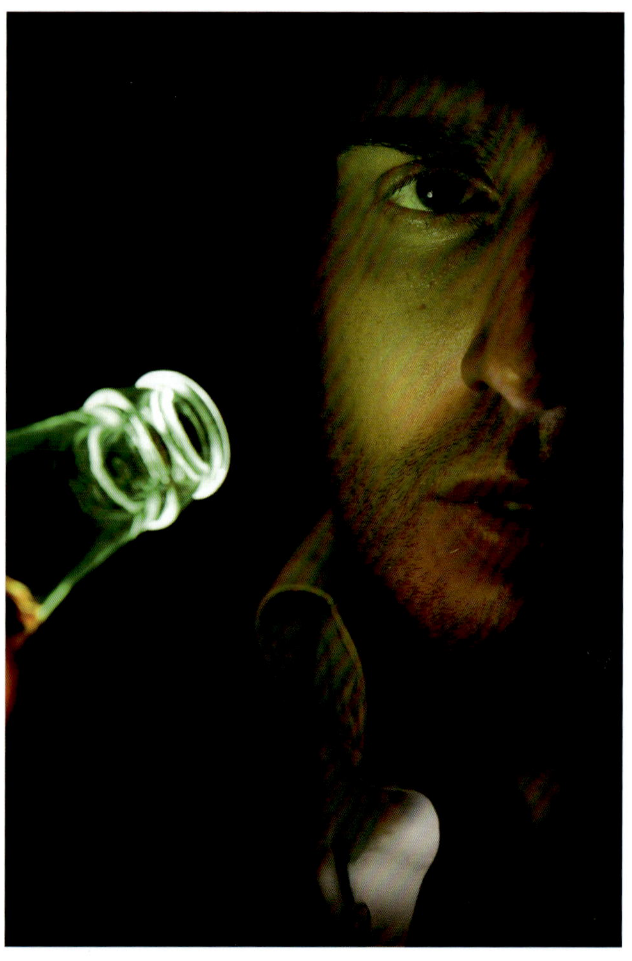

### *3.3.4 Substance misuse among perpetrators*

Caregivers who perpetrate maltreatment against older people are more likely to have mental problems and substance-misuse difficulties than the caregivers with no abusive behaviour *(3,4,24,32,37,43)*. In Ireland, older people reported that 19% of perpetrators misused alcohol *(9)*. Care staff who reported using alcohol to cope with work-related stress were more likely to report being involved in abusive situations, as were family caregivers who used alcohol to relieve stress

*(27)*. Many studies *(24,26,29,44–47)* have found that perpetrators misuse psychoactive substances and are especially alcohol dependent. This has been associated with situations of continued, severe maltreatment and specifically in cases of physical abuse. Perpetrators may thereby develop financial difficulties, which may increase their financial dependence on older relatives.

### *3.3.5 Mental health problems among perpetrators*

Depression is the mental disorder most consistently found among perpetrators of maltreatment among older people *(7,17,18,29,32,41,48,49)*. In Ireland, older people reported that 4% of perpetrators had mental health problems and or intellectual disabilities *(9)*. A study of homicides of older people committed by family members *(12)* found that 54% of perpetrators had some type of mental disorder, with the most common being affective disorders, specifically depression, and psychotic disorders, mainly schizophrenia. Predictive factors for violent behaviour included a prior history of aggressive behaviour, rejection of treatment, thought or perceptual disorders and the consumption of drugs and alcohol *(50)*.

### *3.3.6 Previous history of violent behaviour*

A previous history of violent behaviour is a risk factor. Linked to this are certain mental characteristics such as low impulse control, cognitive distortions, social skills deficits such as in communication and the lack of conflict resolution skills *(50–52)*. Perpetrators may also have problems with social relationships and are more likely to be isolated *(3,4,37)*.

### *3.3.7 Key perpetrator risk factors at the individual level*

The perpetrator risk factors at the individual level that are supported by strong evidence are mental health problems (in particular depression), previous history of violent behaviour and substance misuse, especially alcohol abuse.

## 3.4 Relationship factors

The second level of the ecological model explores how proximal social relationships – such as relations with peers, intimate partners and family members – increase the risk of violent victimization and perpetration of violence *(1)*.

### *3.4.1 Financial dependence of the perpetrator*

In many cases, perpetrators are financially dependent on the victim for their accommodation, maintenance, transport and other costs *(3,4,24,37,46,53–56)*. A study in Spain *(7)* found that the pension of 47% of the older people who were maltreated was the family's main source of income. Financial difficulties among perpetrators are a major risk factor for elder maltreatment *(1,27,55)*. These financial difficulties may sometimes arise due to substance misuse among adult offspring who extort money from their parent to pay for their addiction. Financial abuse of older people may also be triggered by the resentment that family members might feel concerning the costs incurred in caring for the older person *(57)*. In Ireland, more than 50% of perpetrators were not employed at the time that the reported maltreatment occurred *(9)*.

### *3.4.2 Dependence of the perpetrator*

In addition to dependence in financial terms, as seen above, perpetrators may often be highly dependent on their victims for emotional and relational support *(56)*. In addition, in some cases mutual dependence between the victim and the perpetrator was evident and led to the recognition of a web of mutual dependence between the two parties *(56)*. An example from Israel showed increased risk of perpetration by children in multiple-occupancy households in which they were unemployed, financially dependent and had relationship problems *(17)*.

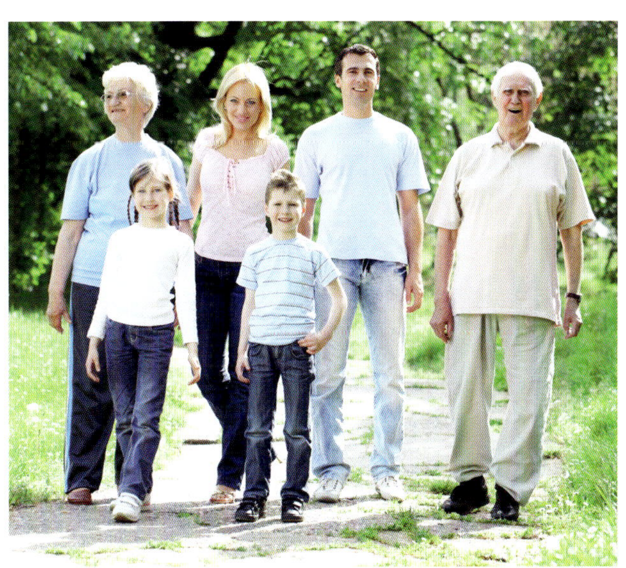

### *3.4.3 Intergenerational transmission of violence*

In some families, violence is a routine and learned behaviour pattern. Family members learn to be violent either through witnessing maltreatment or experiencing it as victims. The family members who have learned to act violently to achieve their goals may replicate this behaviour pattern in their own homes. This behaviour pattern is known as the cycle of violence *(32)*. Few studies have examined this for elder maltreatment, in which little evidence so far indicates intergenerational transmission of violence *(24)*. In Germany, family caregivers reported that poor relationships with the person cared for increased the risk of maltreatment *(27)*. The latest research seems to indicate that the quality of the relationship in general is an important factor, with the type of relationship before the maltreatment occurs possibly being an important predictive factor *(57)*.

### *3.4.4 Shared accommodation*

Interacting on an almost daily basis or sharing living accommodation with a perpetrator may increase the opportunity for violent encounters. Various studies *(11,30,32,58)* show that living alone reduces the risk of maltreatment, whereas living with a family member is a risk factor for becoming a victim of maltreatment. The risk of experiencing maltreatment was greater for people with Alzheimer's disease who lived with close family members *(48)*. Whereas the risk of maltreatment through neglect is minimized when older people live alone, the risk of maltreatment, such as mental and financial abuse, may increase *(8,19)*. The findings from a prevalence study in Israel *(17)* indicated that older people living with partners had an increased risk of maltreatment, including mental abuse. A study in the United Kingdom *(8)* found that people living alone were more likely to report that they had experienced financial abuse in the past year than the participants who were living with other people. The proximity of the perpetrator adversely affects maltreatment (Box 3.2) *(59)*. Some studies *(9,17)* have found that multiple-generation households have the highest levels of maltreatment.

**Box 3.2. Characteristics of the maltreatment that adversely influence how the experience of maltreatment affects the respondents**

Proximity of the perpetrator in terms of relationship and/or living arrangements.

Type and severity of the maltreatment experienced, with more serious maltreatment having more severe impact.

Whether the incident was resolved or not, unresolved situations having greater potential impact on individuals.

Unpredictability of maltreatment and when it might occur, which created more uncertainty and stress for individuals.

Maltreatment that occurred in association with caring responsibilities.

*Source*: Mowlam *(59)*.

### *3.4.5 Kinship of perpetrator to victim*

Most perpetrators were either offspring or a partner *(3,4,11)*. The results of surveys vary, including by types of maltreatment. In Spain, the main perpetrators for older people who are dependent or have disabilities were adult offspring, whereas for independent older people the perpetrators appear to be their partners *(7)*. The study in Ireland identified adult children as the perpetrators (50%), followed by other relatives (24%) or a spouse or partner (20%) *(9)*. Adult children were equally likely to be implicated in financial and other types of abuse, whereas partners were more frequently involved in physical, sexual and mental abuse. Similarly, the prevalence study in Israel found that partners were more likely to perpetrate mental and emotional abuse versus children for financial abuse *(17,18)*. In the ABUEL study, partners were the most frequently reported perpetrators of mental abuse (35%) and physical abuse (34%) and injuries (45%), whereas friends, neighbours and acquaintances were most often reported as perpetrators of sexual abuse (in 30% of cases) *(10)*. A high proportion of intimate partner violence is likely to continue in old age *(37)*. The partners (46%) or children (40%) commit the vast majority of homicides carried out by family members *(12)*. As stated previously, the quality of the relationship before the maltreatment appears to be an important factor *(57)*.

### *3.4.6 Key risk factors at the relationship level*

The risk factors at the relationship level that are supported by strong evidence are the dependence of the perpetrator on the victim (including financial dependence) and shared accommodation for certain types of maltreatment.

## 3.5 Community factors

The third level of the ecological model examines the community contexts – such as care homes, workplaces and neighbourhoods – and seeks to identify the characteristics of these settings that may be associated with being a victim or perpetrator of violence *(1)*. Little information is available on most of these risk factors.

### *3.5.1 Social isolation*

Social isolation is a characteristic risk factor for domestic violence in families *(32)*, and older victims of maltreatment have fewer social contacts *(22,24,31,42,60)*. Whereas older people who reported maltreatment were more likely to be living with someone else (80% in this study), they also have far fewer social ties *(58)*. Victims of elder maltreatment were more likely to have a poor social network and higher levels of social isolation *(22,60)*. The most severe risk to older people may be an abusive situation in social isolation from other family members, friends and welfare agencies or additional forms of community support. This hypothesis needs to be investigated further. Isolation of the family or of individuals is one way of ensuring that the situation remains hidden from the broader society; this may be imposed. Maltreatment is thought to be less likely in the families with strong social networks and connections with society. Available evidence provides broad support for this view. In care homes, lacking family members and having few visitors are associated with more maltreatment *(14)*.

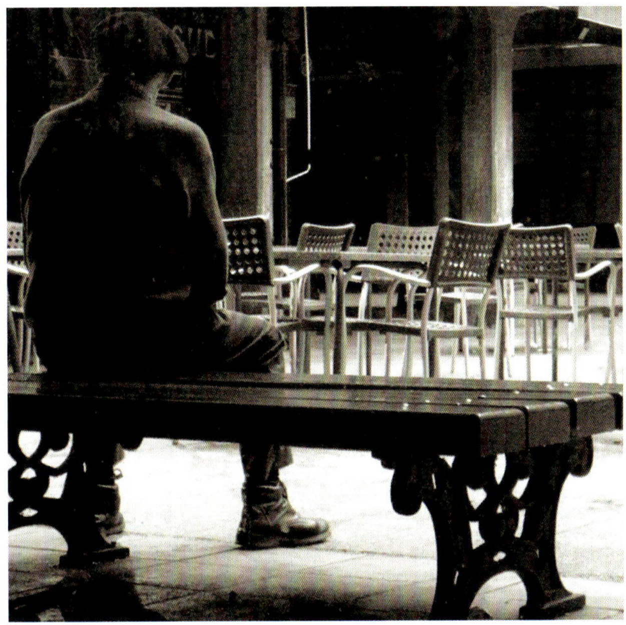

### 3.5.2 Lack of social support

Older people with poor levels of community support were more likely to report maltreatment (physical, sexual and mental abuse) compared with those with strong or moderate levels of community support. Women with poor social support were particularly vulnerable to interpersonal and financial abuse *(9)*. Older people who reported low levels of social support may have higher risks of both mental and financial abuse *(10)*. This suggests that high levels of social support may act as a protective factor and also help to mitigate depressive and anxiety symptoms when maltreatment occurs *(10)*. Older women who were divorced, separated, isolated and lonely were at increased risk of financial abuse compared with others *(8)*.

Many studies show that abusive caregivers lack social support to assist them with their caregiving tasks *(3,4,33,34,37)*. The available data indicate that the importance of lack of social support as a risk factor may be related to the presence of burnout in caregivers, the extremely high levels of need among victims and social isolation, among other factors.

### 3.5.3 Care and health care settings

Maltreatment that occurs in care and health care settings is sometimes referred to as institutional maltreatment. This may relate to institutional policies and practices that operate within such settings. Staff and volunteers may perpetrate maltreatment in these settings but also visitors, whether friends or relatives *(14,61)*. However, even within institutions, much of the maltreatment that takes place happens behind closed doors and is therefore not open to public scrutiny *(62)*.

Little research has examined the nature of risk factors in relation to institutional settings, and much of what is presented is derived from evidence gathered from policy and practice investigations, such as incident inquiries. Box 3.3 summarizes staff characteristics that might play a part in developing or continuing maltreatment; many of these are linked to the institutional setting and may be amenable to targeting with training and resources *(13,14)*. For example, stressful environments increase the risk of staff burnout, which manifests as fatigue and stress and may trigger violent or neglectful acts towards older residents or patients *(14)*.

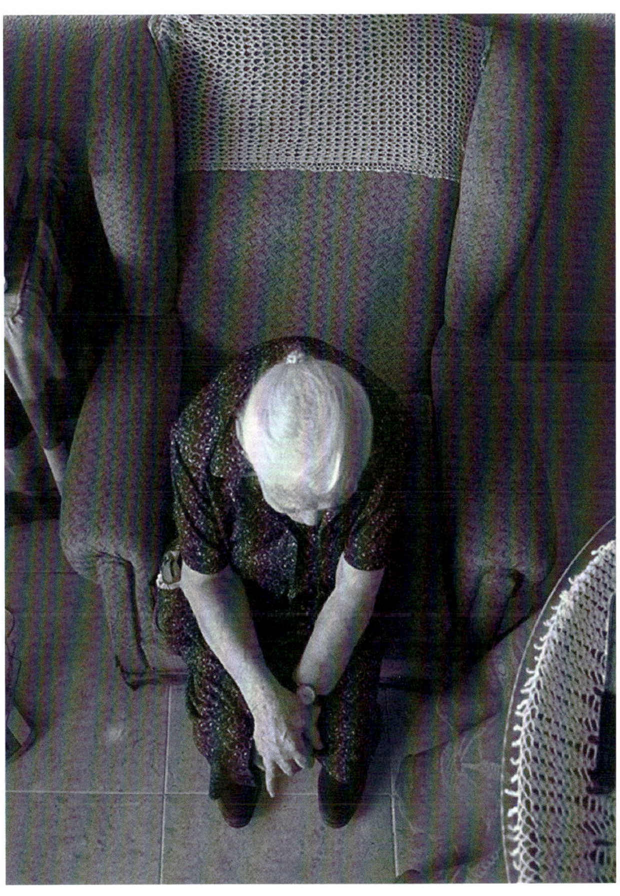

**Box 3.3. Characteristics of staff that are associated with greater maltreatment in care homes**

Lack of qualifications.

Incorrect application of current legislation.

Presence of high stress levels in personal life.

Negative attitudes towards older people.

Low frustration threshold.

Staff burnout.

*Sources*: Juklestad *(13)* and Rubio *(14)*.

Institutional characteristics have been identified as risk factors that relate specifically to the broader level of the institution itself and the care, or lack thereof, provided to older residents *(14,61)*. These include institutions in which the use of aggression is tolerated or condoned, those with poor or inadequate training and support for paid care staff and those with inadequate help available for residents when carrying out daily activities. Further, such institutions may have inflexible routines and regimes, abrupt changes of rooms or environments for residents, with excessive sociocultural activities or infantilization of the older residents, invasion of an older person's privacy and lack of respect.

However, there has been comparatively little research on maltreatment in institutional settings and especially few studies examining risk factors in institutional care. Care homes and hospitals are important for a proportion of older people, especially in the final stages of life, and better research into risk and protective factors is urgently needed.

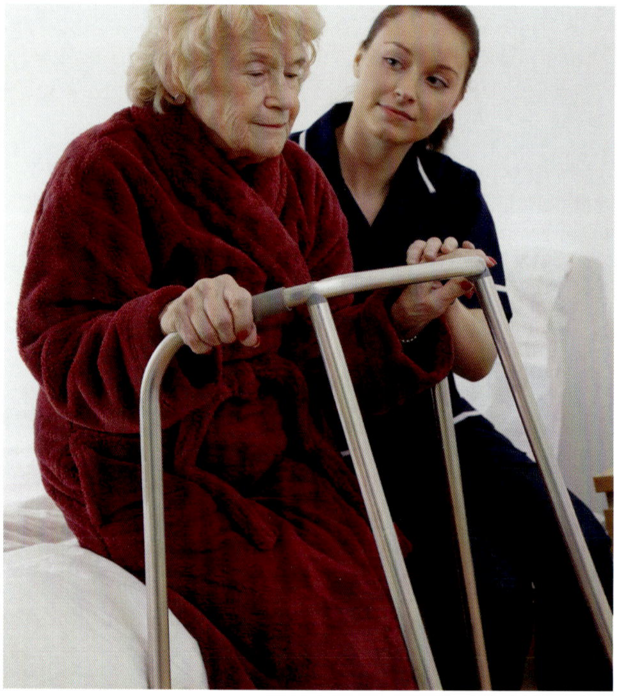

### *3.5.4 Key risk factors at the community level*

The key risk factor at the community level that is supported by strong evidence is social isolation.

## 3.6 Social factors

The fourth level of the ecological model examines the larger societal factors that influence rates of violence. Most of these factors have not been properly studied for elder maltreatment, and more research is needed.

### *3.6.1 Ageism*[12]

Negative attitudes and stereotypes towards older people dehumanize them in various ways. Studies show that both younger generations and the older generation have negative ideas about what old age involves. One perception is that older people lose power and control over their lives with age and become progressively fragile, weak and dependent on other people *(63)*. This makes it easier for other people to maltreat an older person without feeling any guilt or remorse and to see the person as an object for exploitation *(64)*. In this respect, ageism may serve as a societal or cultural backdrop in which elder maltreatment is accepted and permissible *(65)*. It may also mean that attempts to respond to maltreatment and its effects are hindered and made much more difficult to deal with; indeed, the presence of ageism may exacerbate the effects of any maltreatment an individual experiences.

### *3.6.2 Cultural norms supportive of violence*

Cultural and social norms that are tolerant of violence such as attitudes that condone violence as a way of resolving conflict may have an important role in spreading violent behaviour. Other cultures place a higher value on men over women or even see women as men's possessions, condoning violence, and older women may be at greater risk of intimate partner violence *(67)*. The mass media may reflect tolerance of violence in society, and this normalization of violence may contribute to the manifestation of violence. There is concern that such attitudes and beliefs will influence the manifestation of violence towards older people and result in elder maltreatment, although proof is lacking *(68)*.

### *3.6.3 Economic and social factors*

Economic and social policies that influence and maintain high levels of economic and social inequality within societies may add to the tensions that arise between groups. Such factors are likely to play a role in creating a climate in which elder maltreatment is prevalent. Many older people live on low incomes, increasing their dependence on others. Few studies have examined socioeconomic determinants as risk factors for elder maltreatment. In Turkey, a study found that the risk of elder maltreatment increased by more than twice if the educational level was primary school or lower versus secondary school or higher *(69)*. In the United Kingdom, the prevalence of elder maltreatment is reported to be higher among people who had been in routine or semi-routine occupations versus those who had been small employers or self-employed *(8)*. In Israel, educational level was a protective factor for verbal abuse *(17)*. A multi-country study involving seven European countries found that living in rented accommodation as opposed to home ownership appeared to be associated with mental abuse, and having been a homemaker was associated with physical abuse *(10)*. Risk factors for elder maltreatment such as alcohol and drug dependence among perpetrators may be linked to socioeconomic deprivation. Better-designed studies are needed to improve the evidence base for socioeconomic risk determinants.

[12] Robert Butler coined the term ageism in 1969 to refer to "a process by which people are systematically stereotyped for the mere fact of being old, in the same way as racism and sexism act in reaction to the colour of a person's skin or gender" *(66)*.

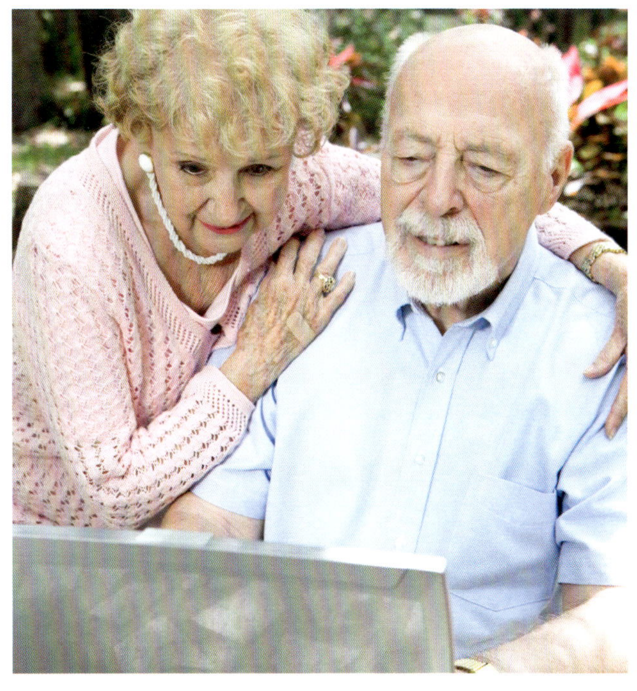

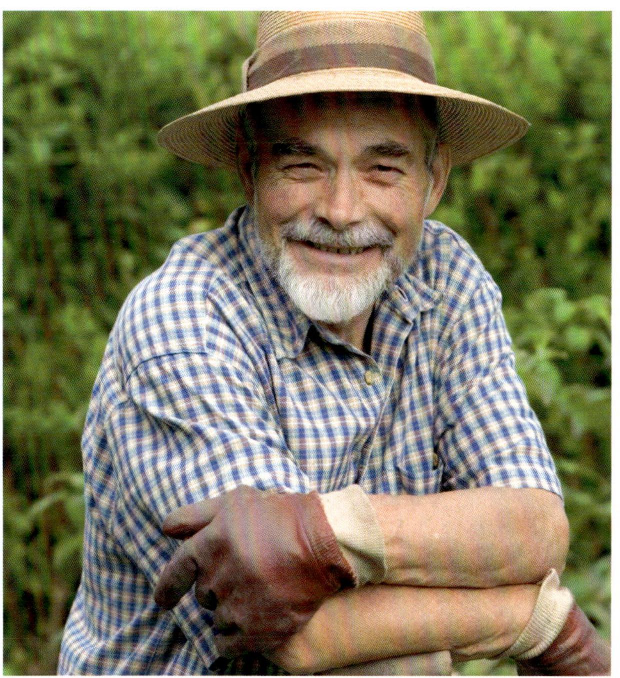

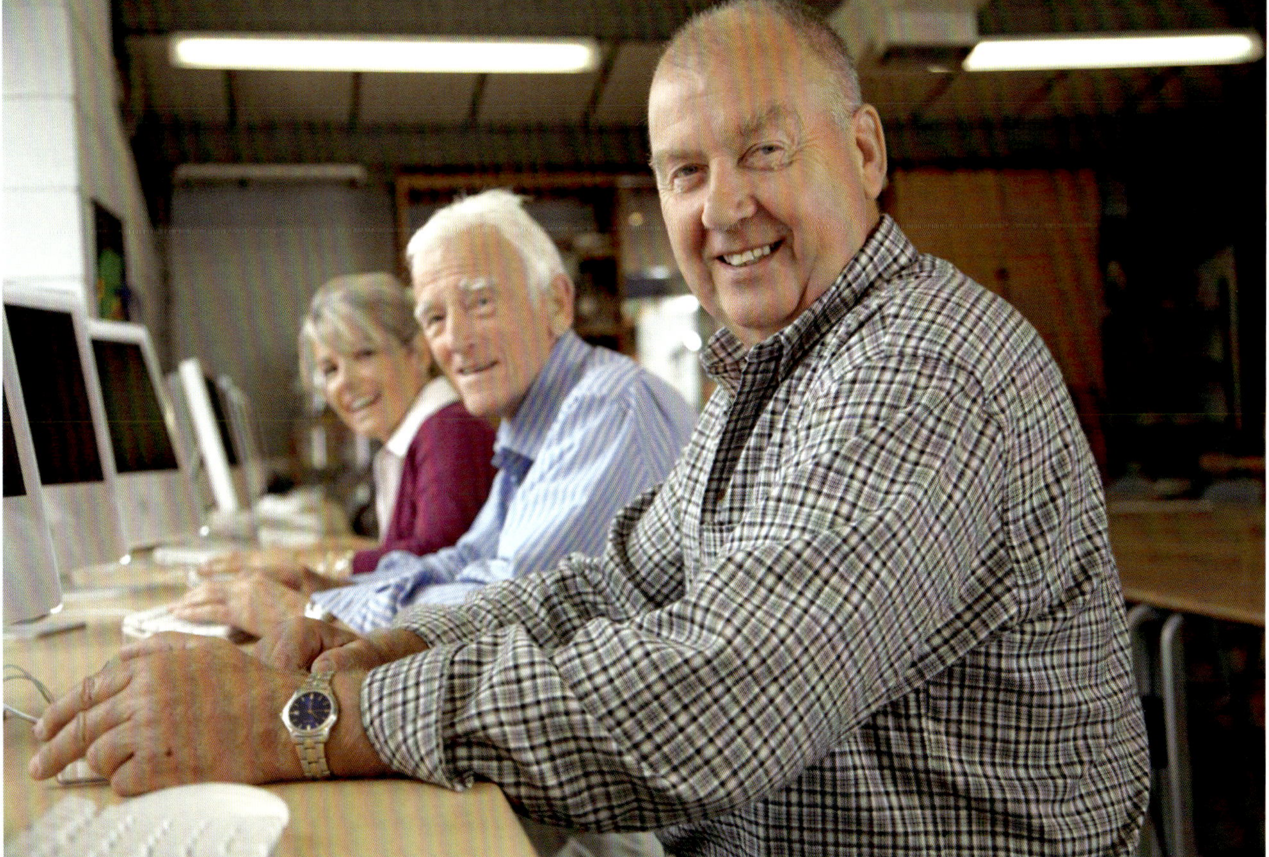

## 3.7 Protective factors helpful to coping with maltreatment

There are protective factors that might assist an individual in withstanding adverse events that might result in elder maltreatment *(70)*.

The study of the prevalence of elder maltreatment in the United Kingdom *(59)* also contained a qualitative element in which individuals who reported maltreatment were interviewed in depth. Factors that were related to the personal circumstances and characteristics of the individual and that might link to both resilience factors and coping mechanisms were identified. This linkage was held to assist in identifying protective factors that may help to prevent or at least ameliorate lasting effects of maltreatment for those who experience such situations. Factors associated with increased resilience to the negative effects of maltreatment or assisting coping mechanisms were identified *(59)*:

- the relationship norms and values of the person, with those reporting more positive relationships and values indicating improved capacity to withstand maltreatment;
- social and community connectedness, with those who were more socially connected reporting less harmful effects of maltreatment;
- religious beliefs, in which individuals with strong beliefs reported that they positively affected their ability to withstand more negative effects;
- living alone, bereavement and fear of being alone as interacting more negatively, so that those who lived alone or were bereaved indicating less resilience to harmful effects;
- health, in which good reported health appeared to strengthen the individual's ability to resist the harmful effects;
- previous life experiences, in which positive prior experiences were a beneficial support;
- personality and personal qualities; and
- specific tactics in the form of coping strategies developed and used to deal with the maltreatment.

However, as indicated, research that examines protective factors is infrequent. In particular, research is needed into protective factors that may mitigate against elder maltreatment from arising in the first place. Such studies should be conducted in both community and other settings.

## 3.8 Synopsis of findings

This chapter has drawn together the available research findings in relation to risk factors for elder maltreatment and presented these within the ecological framework introduced in the first chapter of this report. As acknowledged throughout this chapter, the evidence concerning risk factors is currently somewhat mixed, with strong support from the evidence for some risk factors and contested evidence for other factors, in part because of lack of consistency in identification within the research. In addition, for several risk factors, there is either insufficient evidence or a lack of robust validation of findings from which to draw firm conclusions at this time. Table 3.2 compiles this information and illustrates the strength and importance of risk factors at the various ecological levels from the available evidence.

## 3.9 Summary

The issues that encompass the spectrum of elder maltreatment are complex and multifaceted. Given the nature of the continuum that constitutes the phenomena, any one risk factor is unlikely to be identified as accounting for most maltreatment situations. As stated earlier in this chapter, the reasons maltreatment has occurred and the risk factors involved are likely to be an interaction of several factors, depending on the specific circumstances. Establishing the nature of such factors and exploring the possible interplay between them is therefore important. Although research during the past two decades has provided some insight relating to risk factors, there is still no firm consensus about which risk factors, if any, might be most important and when in developing and continuing situations of elder maltreatment. Indeed, the main limitation noted within much of the research has been a trend until recently to combine all the forms of maltreatment *(71)*, so that determining discrete risk factors for the various types of maltreatment remains difficult.

Evidence is partial for such factors as gender, race and the relationship of the victim to the perpetrator or even contested for such factors as physical impairment of the victim, dependence of the victim, caregiver stress and the intergenerational transmission of maltreatment. Nevertheless, strong evidence implicates the following risk factors: social isolation, living arrangements, dementia, intraindividual characteristics of the perpetrators such as mental illness, high levels of hostility and alcohol abuse and dependence of the perpetrator on the victim.

### Key messages

Recent high-quality research studies of the risk factors related to elder maltreatment are lacking, both within the European Region and elsewhere, creating difficulty in drawing firm conclusions on risk factors.

The cycles of violence need to be addressed to reduce perpetration by those who were once victims.

Strong evidence implicates the following risk factors: social isolation, living arrangements, dementia, intraindividual characteristics of perpetrators such as mental ill health, hostility and alcohol abuse and dependence of the perpetrator on the victim.

There has also been a general lack of research examining protective factors that strengthen individuals' abilities to withstand the harmful effects of elder maltreatment.

Wherever possible, research should be undertaken using robust methods that address risk and protective factors and includes the outcomes of elder maltreatment.

Further research is needed to fully determine the most important risk and protective factors at different levels of the ecological model. This would assist in developing and targeting strategies to prevent and intervene in situations of elder maltreatment.

**Table 3.2. Risk factors identified and strength of the evidence**

| Level | Main risk factors | Strength of the evidence |
|---|---|---|
| Individual (victim) | Sex: women | Potential |
| | Age: older than 74 years | Contested |
| | Dependence: high levels of physical or intellectual disability | Contested |
| | Dementia, including Alzheimer's disease and other types of dementia | Strong |
| | Mental disorders: depression | Potential |
| | Aggression and challenging behaviour by the victim | Potential |
| Individual (perpetrator) | Sex: men in cases of physical abuse and women in neglect cases | Potential |
| | Mental disorders: depression | Strong |
| | Substance abuse: alcohol and drug misuse | Strong |
| | Hostility and aggression | Strong |
| | Financial problems | Strong |
| | Stress: caregiver burnout | Contested |
| Relationship | Financial dependence of the perpetrator on the victim | Strong |
| | Dependence of the perpetrator on the victim (emotional and accommodation) | Strong |
| | Intergenerational transmission of violence | Contested |
| | Long-term history of difficulty in the relationship | Potential |
| | Kinship: children or partner | Potential |
| | Living arrangement | Strong |
| Community | Social isolation: victim lives alone with perpetrator and both have few social contacts | Strong |
| | Lack of social support: absence of social support resources and systems | Potential |
| Societal | Discrimination due to age: ageism | Potential |
| | Other forms of discrimination: sexism and racism | Potential |
| | Social and economic factors | Potential |
| | Violent culture: normalization of violence | Potential |

In situations involving maltreatment or neglect of older people or even when older people face difficult and problematic situations in which maltreatment has not yet happened, risk factors are clearly of high importance. However, identifying risk factors within situations involving older people does not necessarily indicate that maltreatment is definitely taking place or will occur. Recognizing the relevant risk factors within such situations should instead heighten awareness of the possibility that the situation may be (or may become) abusive so that appropriate further investigation and enquiries can take place and suitable responses offered as necessary. In addition, addressing and reducing risk factors to help prevent elder maltreatment from occurring are important. Risk factors have a key role to play, therefore, in both preventing and intervention in elder maltreatment. This is likely to be of increasing significance given the growing societal awareness of elder maltreatment and the greater emphasis on assessing and managing the risk of abusive situations. The evidence base relating to such matters therefore needs to be revised as necessary following additional research, and strategies for prevention, including promoting protective factors, and intervention need to be regularly updated to reflect any changes required.

## 3.10 References


1. Krug E et al., eds. *World report on violence and health*. Geneva, World Health Organization, 2002 (http://www.who.int/violence_injury_prevention/violence/world_report/en, accessed 9 May 2011).

2. Bonnie R, Wallace R, eds. *Elder mistreatment: abuse, neglect, and exploitation in an aging America*. Washington, DC, National Academies Press, 2003.

3. Cooney C, Mortimer A. Elder abuse and dementia: a pilot study. *International Journal of Social Psychiatry*, 1995, 4:276–283.

4. González JA et al. Malos tratos al anciano [Elder maltreatment]. In: Sánchez T, ed. *Maltrato de género, infantil y de ancianos [Gender-based maltreatment and maltreatment of children and older people]*. Salamanca, Publicaciones Universidad Pontificia de Salamanca, 2005:105–119 (Temas de psicología X).

5. Wolf R. Elder abuse and neglect: causes and consequences. *Journal of Geriatric Psychiatry*, 1997, 30:153–174.

6. Iborra I. Maltrato de personas mayors [Elder maltreatment]. *Diario de Campo*, 2006, Suppl. 40:53–60.

7. Iborra I. *Maltrato de personas mayores en la familia en España [Elder maltreatment within families in Spain]*. Valencia, Queen Sofía Center, 2008 (Serie Documentos No. 13).

8. O'Keeffe M et al. *The UK study of abuse and neglect of older people*. London, National Centre for Social Research, 2007.

9. Naughton C et al. *Abuse and neglect of older people in Ireland. Report on the National Study of Elder Abuse and Neglect*. Dublin, National Centre for the Protection of Older People, 2010.

10. Soares JJF et al. *Abuse and health in Europe*. Kaunas, Lithuanian University of Health Sciences Press, 2010.

11. Pillemer K, Finkelhor D. The prevalence of elder abuse: a random sample survey. *The Gerontologist*, 1988, 28:51–57.

12. Iborra I, Sanmartín J, López MJ. *Ancianos asesinados por familiares en España [Homicide victims among older people perpetrated by family members in Spain]*. Valencia, Queen Sofía Center, in press.

13. Juklestad O. Institutional care for older people – the dark side. *Journal of Adult Protection*, 2001, 3(2):32–41.

14. Rubio R. Concepto, tipos, incidencia y factores de riesgo del maltrato institucional de personas mayores [Concept, types, incidence and risk factors for institutional elder maltreatment]. In: Iborra I, ed. *Violencia contra personas mayores [Violence against older people]*. Barcelona, Editorial Ariel, 2005 (Colección Estudios sobre Violencia, No. 11).

15. *Hidden voices: older people's experience of abuse*. Streatham, Action on Elder Abuse and Help the Aged, 2005.

16. *The National Elder Abuse Incidence Study*. New York, National Center on Elder Abuse, 1998.

17. Lowenstein A, Eisikovits Z, Winterstein T. Is elder abuse and neglect a social phenomenon? Data from the first national prevalence survey in Israel. *Journal of Elder Abuse and Neglect*, 2009, 21:253–277.

18. Siegel-Itzkovich J. A fifth of elderly people in Israel are abused. *British Medical Journal*, 2005, 330:498.

19. Garre-Olmo J et al. Prevalence and risk factors of suspected elder abuse subtypes in people aged 75 and older. *Journal of the American Geriatrics Society*, 2009, 57:815–822.

20. Davidson JL. Elder abuse. In: Block MR, Sinnott JD, eds. *The battered elder syndrome: an exploratory study*. College Park, MD, Center on Aging, University of Maryland, 1979:239–252.

21. Hickey T, Douglass RL. Mistreatment of the elderly in the domestic setting: an exploratory study. *American Journal of Public Health*, 1981, 71:500–507.

22. Lachs MS et al. A prospective community-based pilot study of risk factors for the investigation of elder mistreatment. *Journal of the American Geriatrics Society*, 1994, 42:169–173.

23. Steinmetz SK. *Duty bound: elder abuse and family care*. Newbury Park, CA, Sage Publications, 1988.

24. Wolf R, Pillemer K. *Helping elderly victims: the reality of elder abuse*. New York, Columbia University Press, 1989.

25. Yan ECW, Tang CSK. Elder abuse by caregivers: a study of prevalence and risk factors in Hong Kong

Chinese families. *Journal of Family Violence*, 2004, 19:269–277.

26. Perez-Carceles MD et al. Suspicion of elder abuse in south eastern Spain: the extent and risk factors. *Archives of Gerontology and Geriatrics*, 2009, 49:132–137.

27. Görgen T et al. *Kriminalitäts- und Gewaltgefährdungen im Leben älterer Menschen – Zusammenfassung wesentlicher Ergebnisse einer Studie zu Gefährdungen älterer und pflegebedürftiger Menschen [Experiences of crime and violence in older people's lives: summary of the key results of a study on hazards to older people and care recipients]*. Berlin, Federal Ministry of Family Affairs, Senior Citizens, Women and Youth, 2009.

28. Bazo MT. Diversas manifestaciones de la violencia familiar [Various types of family violence]. *Alternativas Cuadernos de Trabajo Social*, 2002, 10:213–219.

29. Homer AC. Gilleard C. Abuse of elderly people by their carers. *British Medical Journal*, 1990, 301:1359–1362.

30. Pillemer K, Suitor J. Violence and violent feelings: what causes them among family caregivers. *Journal of Gerontology*, 1992, 47:S165–S172.

31. Compton SA, Flanagan P, Gregg W. Elder abuse in people with dementia in Northern Ireland: prevalence and predictors in cases referred to a psychiatry of old age service. *International Journal of Geriatric Psychiatry*, 1997, 12:632–635.

32. Pillemer K. Factores de riesgo del maltrato de mayores [Risk factors in elder maltreatment]. In: Iborra I, ed. *Violencia contra personas mayores [Violence against older people]*. Barcelona, Ariel, 2005:69–85.

33. Perez-Rojo G et al. Identification of elder abuse risk factors in community settings. *International Journal of Clinical and Health Psychology*, 2008, 8:105–117.

34. Perez-Rojo G et al. Risk factors of elder abuse in a community dwelling Spanish sample. *Archives of Gerontology and Geriatrics*, 2009, 49:17–21.

35. Comijs HC et al. Elder abuse in the community: prevalence and consequences. *Journal of the American Geriatrics Society*, 1998, 46:885–888.

36. O'Loughlin A, Duggan J. *Abuse, neglect and mistreatment of older people: an exploratory study*. Dublin, National Council on Ageing and Older People, 1998 (Report No. 52).

37. Muñoz J. *Personas mayores y malos tratos [Older people and maltreatment]*. Madrid, Ediciones Pirámide, 2004.

38. Iborra I. Incidencia y prevalencia del maltrato de mayores [Incidence and prevalence of elder maltreatment]. In: Iborra I, ed. *Violencia contra personas mayores [Violence against older people]*. Barcelona, Editorial Ariel, 2005 (Colección Estudios sobre Violencia, No. 11).

39. Biggs S et al. Mistreatment of the older people in the United Kingdom: findings from the first National Prevalence Study. *Journal of Elder Abuse and Neglect*, 2009, 21:1–14.

40. Freudenberger HJ. Staff burnout. *Journal of Social Issues*, 1974, 30:159–165.

41. Coyne A, Reichman W. The relationship between dementia and elder abuse. *American Journal of Psychiatry*, 1993, 150:643–646.

42. Grafstrom M, Nordberg A, Winblad B. Abuse is in the eye of the beholder. *Scandinavian Journal of Social Medicine*, 1993, 21:247–255.

43. Lachs MS, Pillemer K. Abuse and neglect of elderly persons. *New England Journal of Medicine*, 1995, 332:437–443.

44. Anetzberger GJ, Korbin JE, Austin C. Alcoholism and elder abuse. *Journal of Interpersonal Violence*, 1994, 9:184–193.

45. Bristowe E, Collins JB. Family mediated abuse of non-institutionalized frail elderly men and women living in British Columbia. *Journal of Elder Abuse and Neglect*, 1989, 1:45–64.

46. Greenberg JR, McKibben M, Raymond JA. Dependent adult children and elder abuse. *Journal of Elder Abuse and Neglect*, 1990, 2:73–86.

47. Reay AM, Browne KD. Risk factor characteristics in carers who physically abuse or neglect their elderly dependants. *Ageing and Mental Health*, 2001, 5:56–62.

48. Paveza GJ et al. Severe family violence and Alzheimer's disease: prevalence and risk factors. *The Gerontologist*, 1992, 32:493–497.

49. Williamson GM, Shaffer DR. Relationship quality and potentially harmful behaviors by spousal caregivers:

how we were then, how we are now. *Psychology and Aging*, 2001, 16:217–226.

50. Echeburúa E et al. ¿Se puede y debe tratar psicológicamente a los hombres violentos contra la pareja? [Can and should men who carry out intimate partner violence receive psychological treatment?] *Papeles del Psicólogo*, 2004, 88:20–28.

51. Corral P. Perfil del agresor doméstico [Profile of people who carry out domestic violence]. In: Sanmartín J, ed. *El laberinto de la violencia. Causas, tipos y efectos [The labyrinth of violence. Causes, types and effects]*. Barcelona, Ariel, 2004 (Colección Estudios sobre Violencia, No. 10).

52. Echeburúa E, Fernández-Montalvo J, Amor PJ. Psychopathological profile of men convicted of gender violence: a study in the prisons of Spain. *Journal of Interpersonal Violence*, 2003, 18:798–812.

53. Anetzberger GJ. *The etiology of elder abuse by adult offspring.* Springfield, IL, Charles C. Thomas, 1983.

54. Hwalek MA, Sengstock MC, Lawrence R. Assessing the probability of abuse of the elderly. *37th Annual Scientific Meeting of the Gerontological Society of America, San Antonio, TX, USA, 16–20 November 1984*.

55. Pillemer KA. Risk factors in elder abuse: results from a case-control study. In: Pillemer KA, Wolf RS, eds. *Elder abuse: conflict in the family*. Dover, Auburn House Publishing Company, 1986:239–263.

56. Wolf RS, Strugnell CP, Godkin MA. *Preliminary findings from three model projects on elderly abuse*. Worcester, MA, University of Massachusetts Medical Center on Aging, 1982.

57. Wolf R, Daichman L, Bennett G. Abuse of the elderly. In: Krug E et al., eds. *World report on violence and health*. Geneva, World Health Organization, 2002:123–146 (http://www.who.int/violence_injury_prevention/violence/world_report/en, accessed 9 May 2011).

58. Lachs MS et al. Risk factors for reported elder abuse and neglect: a nine-year observational cohort study. *The Gerontologist*, 1997, 37:469–474.

59. Mowlam A et al. *UK Study of Abuse and Neglect of Older People: qualitative findings.* London, National Centre for Social Research, 2007.

60. Phillips RL. Abuse and neglect of the frail elderly at home: an exploration of theoretical relationships. *Journal of Advanced Nursing*, 1983, 8:379–392.

61. Gilleard C. Physical abuse in homes and hospitals. In: Eastman M, ed. *Old age abuse: a new perspective*. London, Age Concern, 1994.

62. Bennett G, Kingston P, Penhale B. *The dimensions of elder abuse: perspectives for practitioners.* Basingstoke, Macmillan, 1997.

63. *Percepciones sociales sobre las personas mayors [Social perceptions of older people]*. Madrid, Institute of Migration and Social Services, Ministry of Labour and Social Affairs, 2002.

64. Bytheway B. *Ageism*. Buckingham, Open University Press, 1994.

65. Penhale B, Parke J, Kingston P. *Elder abuse: approaches to working with violence*. Birmingham, BASW/Venture Press, 2000.

66. Johnson J, Bytheway B. Ageism: concept and definition. In: Johnson J, Slater R, eds. *Ageing and later life*. London, Sage Publications, 1993.

67. Sanmartín J. *El enemigo en casa. La violencia familiar [The enemy at home. Family violence]*. Barcelona, Nabla ediciones, 2008.

68. Browne K. Family violence: spouse and elder abuse. In: Howells K. Hollin CR, eds. *Clinical approaches to violence*. Chichester, Wiley, 1989.

69. Kissal A, Beser A. Elder abuse and neglect in a population offering care by a primary health care center in Izmir, Turkey. *Social Work in Health Care*, 2011, 50:158–175.

70. Kazdin AE et al. Contributions of risk-factor research to developmental psychopathology. *Clinical Psychology Review*, 1997, 17:375–406.

71. Penhale B. Responding and intervening in elder abuse. *Ageing International*, 2010, 35:235–232.

# 4. Interventions to prevent and reduce elder maltreatment

## 4.1 Introduction

Preventing and reducing elder maltreatment requires implementing evidence-based interventions and programmes. This requires a good understanding of the types of intervention that offer potential for prevention, the beneficial and sometimes adverse effects each approach has on victims, perpetrators and professionals and the costs associated with implementation. Numerous interventions have been put into place to address elder maltreatment both across the European Region and elsewhere. This chapter explores these interventions, highlights examples from across the European Region where possible and discusses the strength of evidence to support their use. Table 4.1 summarizes evidence for interventions to prevent and reduce elder maltreatment.

Although this chapter mainly focuses on interventions specifically designed to address elder maltreatment, there have been very few high-quality evaluations of such programmes so far. Two comprehensive reviews of interventions to prevent elder maltreatment *(1,2)* emphasize the need for more high-quality research and conclude that insufficient evidence currently supports the effectiveness of any one programme. This chapter therefore aims to present a broader perspective, including interventions that aim to reduce risk factors for maltreatment (such as caregiver stress, lack of social support for caregivers and ageism; see Chapter 3). Although they have not been included, more general strategies for preventing violence are also likely to be important in preventing elder maltreatment. These approaches aim to create safe, stable and nurturing relationships between individuals (particularly infants and parents or caregivers) and to develop the life and social skills needed to successfully navigate and deal with everyday life *(3,4)*.

The chapter is structured according to intervention target populations at different levels: universal approaches target the general population or are implemented across the whole of a group of individuals (such as for all health care personnel); selective approaches target individuals at risk of elder maltreatment (either as victims or perpetrators); and indicated approaches target the victims or perpetrators of maltreatment. Since some interventions do not fit neatly within any of the above categories, a fourth and fifth category are included: organizational interventions (those designed to improve professional practice through for instance guidance and protocols) and multicomponent interventions.

### Key facts

High-quality evaluation studies of interventions specifically designed to reduce elder maltreatment are lacking, both within the European Region and elsewhere. This substantially limits conclusions about which interventions may be most effective in reducing or preventing elder maltreatment.

There are mixed findings for the effectiveness of professional awareness and education courses; legal, psychological and educational support programmes and restraint reduction programmes in reducing elder maltreatment. More research is needed to clarify the effects.

Evidence of effectiveness (from just one high-quality study) is emerging for psychological programmes for people who maltreat, which have been associated with a reduction in self-reported maltreatment behaviour. However, further high-quality evaluations of these programmes are needed to provide better understanding of potential effects.

There is some promising evidence for the use of programmes designed to change attitudes towards older people or improve caregiver mental health, but effects on elder maltreatment have not yet been measured.

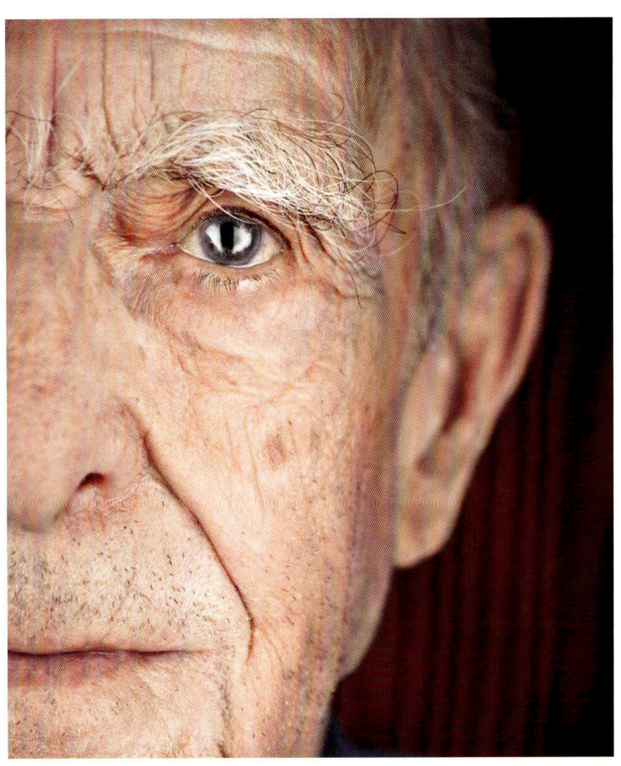

**Table 4.1. Summary of evidence for interventions to prevent and reduce elder maltreatment**

| Intervention | | Impact | |
|---|---|---|---|
| | | **Impact on elder maltreatment** | **Impact on risk factors for elder maltreatment** |
| **Universal** | Public information campaigns | No studies | |
| | Professional awareness and education | Mixed or unclear findings | |
| | School-based intergenerational programmes | | Promising evidence (improvement in positive attitudes towards older people) |
| **Selective** | Screening | No studies | |
| | Education campaigns for older people | No studies | |
| | Caregiver education programmes | No studies | |
| | Encouraging positive attitudes among those working with older people | | Promising evidence (improvement in positive attitudes towards older people) |
| | Informal caregiver support programmes | | Promising evidence (reduction in caregiver burden, stress and depression) |
| **Indicated** | Adult protective services | No studies | |
| | Legal, psychological and educational support | Mixed or unclear findings | |
| | Helplines | No studies | |
| | Emergency shelters | No studies | |
| | Psychological programmes for people who maltreat | Emerging evidence (decline in self-reported maltreatment behaviour) | |
| | Restraint reduction programmes | Mixed or unclear findings | |
| **Other** | Organizational interventions | No studies | |
| | Multicomponent interventions | No studies | |

No studies: no higher-quality evaluation studies. Higher-quality studies have been defined as those using a quantitative design, including a control group for comparison and using a sample likely to be representative of the target population.
Mixed or unclear findings: higher-quality evaluation studies report mixed or unclear findings.
Emerging evidence: evidence of an effect from one higher-quality evaluation study only; more high-quality research is needed to clarify the effects reported.
Promising evidence: evidence of an effect from several higher-quality evaluation studies.

## 4.2 Universal approaches

### *4.2.1 Public information campaigns*

Public information campaigns aim to raise awareness of elder maltreatment across society through the use of such mass media as television, radio, printed materials and web sites. Although the focus differs between campaigns, they often provide or encourage: education about available support services; positive attitudes towards older people; action to prevent and reduce maltreatment; and respectful, dignified treatment of older people. Numerous examples of elder maltreatment campaigns can be found throughout the European Region (Box 4.1 provides examples). Although such campaigns are one of the most visible interventions for addressing maltreatment, they are notoriously difficult to evaluate scientifically. Consequently, there are no known higher-quality[13] evaluations of campaigns evaluating effects on understanding and awareness of elder maltreatment, levels of maltreatment, or levels of reporting. Nevertheless, the use of mass media might help to turn an often hidden and neglected problem into something more noticeable and less tolerable within society. Raising awareness of maltreatment and challenging negative societal attitudes towards older people are both important steps to developing effective protection against elder maltreatment.

**Box 4.1. Some examples of elder maltreatment campaigns within the WHO European Region**

United Kingdom
Help the Aged launched the Enough is Enough campaign in 2007 to raise awareness of elder maltreatment across society. In particular, the campaign aimed to dispel the myth that maltreatment of older people is only a problem within institutions. Information booklets were distributed alongside the campaign that highlighted the main signs of maltreatment and the steps that could be taken to help prevent it.

Spain
Ponte en su Piel (Put Yourself in Their Skin) is an Internet-based campaign seeking to raise awareness of elder maltreatment. Launched in 2002, it promotes a decalogue against elder maltreatment: 10 ways to protect against elder maltreatment and provide better quality care. The campaign encourages businesses, services and individuals to include the decalogue within protocols and culture.

Ireland
A national campaign entitled Open Your Eyes was launched in 2008–2009 to raise awareness and understanding of elder maltreatment among the general public (targeted at those aged 50 years or over). The campaign was run over three separate weeks over the course of two months. It involved radio and television advertising and the distribution of information leaflets on elder maltreatment (including the promotion of a helpline for those requiring additional support). In addition, articles were published and press releases launched to create public discussion around elder maltreatment *(5)*.

[13] This report defines higher-quality studies as those using a quantitative design, including a control group for comparison and using a sample likely to be representative of the target population.

### *4.2.2 Professional awareness and education courses*

Social and health care professionals who come into routine contact with older people are in an ideal position to identify and support those at risk of or already experiencing maltreatment. Training and education programmes aim to increase professional awareness of elder maltreatment and improve professionals' ability to identify and deal effectively with suspected cases; they are considered essential in improving the protection of older adults. Education courses on elder maltreatment often form part of routine training for health and social care professionals. Although they vary in content, they typically include: education about the signs and symptoms of elder maltreatment; discussion around the roles and responsibilities of professionals in protecting older people; discussion of ethical issues around reporting; training in problem-solving skills; training in evaluation and assessment; and training in strategies to manage cases effectively. Programmes have been delivered through workshops (Box 4.2) *(6,7)*, formal training courses (Box 4.2) *(2,9)*, home visiting *(10,11)* and online *(12)* or printed *(9)* learning materials.

Although there have been numerous evaluations of training and education programmes, these have varied substantially in quality. The higher-quality evaluations *(9,11)* have mixed results. In the United Kingdom, an educational intervention for nurses, care assistants and social workers was implemented using two delivery formats: a formal educational course and printed educational material *(9)*. Although no improvements in professional knowledge and management of elder maltreatment were reported for those given printed materials, improvements were noted for professionals on the educational course, especially those with lower baseline knowledge. Conversely, in the United States, a home visiting programme for family practice residency graduates involved three-year geriatric rotations to evaluate potential victims of elder maltreatment. After controlling for confounding factors, there were no differences compared with a comparison group on graduates' reported comfort in diagnosing maltreatment. Further, the percentages of graduates and controls identifying maltreatment did not differ *(11)*.

Drawing any firm conclusions from the available studies is difficult, but it would appear that: the format of delivery (such as an education course or printed material) is important for effectiveness; interventions may prove more effective if they involve those with lower baseline knowledge about elder maltreatment; and more research is needed to clarify the potentially beneficial short-term effects of the interventions. Essentially, however, little is known about the effectiveness of education and training programmes in reducing the likelihood of elder maltreatment (that is, little is known about what happens once a suspected case has been identified). This is particularly important, since the outcomes of interventions for victims of maltreatment appear to be mixed and, in some instances, subsequent levels of maltreatment may even increase (see subsection 4.4.1.2). Thus, the effectiveness of education and training programmes for professionals also largely depends on the strategies put in place to deal with a suspected case once it is identified.

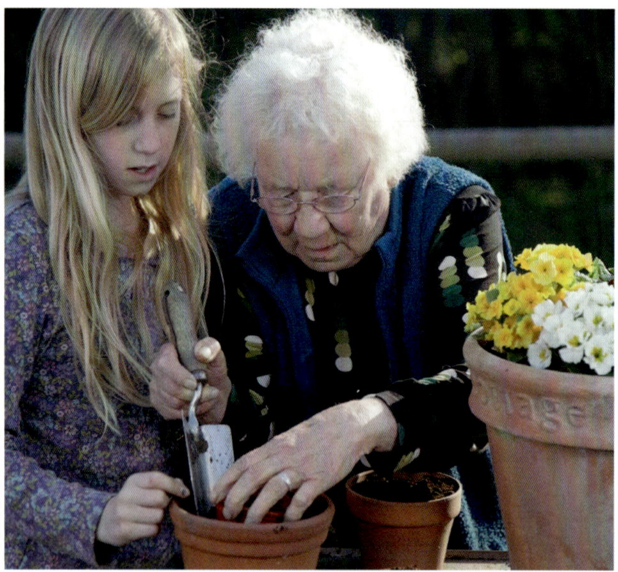

### *4.2.3 Intergenerational programmes*

Negative societal attitudes and stereotypes towards older people may make elder maltreatment and neglect more tolerable within society and of low perceived importance (Chapter 3) *(13)*. For instance, older people may be less valued within societies that perceive them to be frail, weak and dependent or to have diminished physical and mental abilities. One approach used to encourage positive attitudes towards older people is to offer opportunities for meaningful interaction between older adults and young people by using intergenerational programmes. Such programmes aim to influence not only personal attitudes but also, through group discussion and interaction, social attitudes and stereotypes.

Intergenerational programmes allow different age groups to learn about each other and to dispel any misconceived stereotypes. Programmes often target school or university students *(14–16)* but may also involve youths from community settings (such as through church groups *(17)*, summer camps *(18)* or employment programmes *(18)*). Programmes vary in the extent of interaction between the two age groups and the type of activities completed *(19)*. For instance, simple intergenerational programmes involve only indirect contact through exchanging letters or e-mails. More engaging programmes involve direct contact through visiting local nursing homes, sharing group activities such as solving problems, creative activities or playing games, participation in joint community projects or help with everyday life (such as a young person providing house or garden care and an older person offering individual tutoring).

Programme evaluations have often been small in scale, conducted in the United States and involving older children (ages 8–12 years). The higher-quality evaluations provide evidence that the programmes can significantly improve attitudes among participants compared with control groups, at least in the short term *(14,15,20–24)*. However, little is known about whether these changes are sustained in the longer term, whether they have any wider effects on social perceptions and stereotypes of older people or whether such a change in attitudes early on in life would protect against the subsequent perpetration of elder maltreatment.

**Box 4.2. Examples of professional awareness and education courses within the WHO European Region**

Germany

The German Police University in Münster runs Sicher leben im Alter (secure life in old age). Home care nurses and middle managers are educated in identifying maltreatment and intervening in a professional manner. The project works at the individual (nurses) and organizational (home care services) levels. Delivered using workshops and formal courses, the programme includes: information on elder maltreatment; risk factors; screening; communication in critical care situations; and legal issues. The project started in late 2008 and will finish in 2011.

Ireland

A workshop on elder maltreatment and self-neglect has been developed for social work and public health nursing students to increase awareness of maltreatment and prepare them for their role in safeguarding vulnerable older people. The workshop is delivered in two sessions (six hours in total) and uses a variety of methods such as presentations, online reading resources, discussions and case studies. Topics covered include: definitions of maltreatment; prevalence; risk factors; policy; legislation; assessment tools; and possible interventions *(6)*.

Multiple countries

Breaking the Taboo Two is a collaborative project involving several countries (Austria, Finland, Belgium, Bulgaria, Germany, Portugal and Slovenia). The project aims to raise awareness of violence against older women in families and to empower health and social service professionals to recognize abusive situations and to intervene. Part of the project involves developing a curriculum to educate health and social service professionals, especially those involved in home care. The project is due to end in December 2011.

## 4.3 Selective approaches

### *4.3.1 Involving potential victims*

*4.3.1.1 Screening*

Improving the identification of the people at risk of maltreatment can help ensure that victims and potential victims access appropriate social, medical, psychological and legal support needed to improve their situations. Health professionals often use screening tools to aid in identifying maltreatment among patients. These comprise a short series of questions that enquire about recent behaviour and experiences to help to assess whether maltreatment is occurring or is likely to occur. Possible signs of maltreatment include having: cognitive impairment, a history of past maltreatment, problems with alcohol use, conflicts with family members, excessively demanding behaviour or suspicious falls or injuries *(25)*. Screening tools that have been found to be reliable and/or valid include the Elder Abuse Suspicion Index *(26)*, the Indicators of Abuse screen *(25,27)* and the Elders Psychological Abuse Scale *(28)*. Studies comparing methods of delivering questions suggest that telephone interviews can be acceptable among older people and effective in detecting maltreatment compared with face-to-face interviews *(29)*. Further, older people may use new technologies such as computer-assisted personal interviews or computer-assisted telephone interviews, which may be effective in increasing reporting of maltreatment *(30)*.

Studies evaluating the use of screening tools in practice are rare, and no higher-quality evaluations have explored effects on either referral to support services or longer-term elder maltreatment outcomes. However, as with professional awareness and education courses (subsection 4.2.2), the effectiveness of screening inevitably depends on the programmes and interventions put in place once an older person has been identified as being at risk of or experiencing maltreatment (see section 4.4). Further, several concerns have been raised about the use of screening tools among health professionals. These include: the possibility of detecting false positives; the possibility of abusive caregivers being present at professional appointments (providing little opportunity to complete screening tools in private); and ethical concerns around reporting maltreatment if suspected *(2)*. In particular, whistle-blowers may fear reprisal or victimization from an employer if the perpetrator reported is a colleague (Box 4.3).

*4.3.1.2 Educational campaigns for potential victims of elder maltreatment*

Increasing awareness of elder maltreatment and the available support is important not only for the general public (subsection 4.2.1) and health professionals (subsection 4.2.2), but also among the people at risk of experiencing maltreatment. Educational campaigns have been developed that target older people specifically and aim to increase awareness of acceptable and unacceptable caregiving behaviour and available support services. For instance, in Canada, a mass-media campaign was developed and disseminated to older people via newspapers, television and radio, along with leaflets in pharmacies, meals-on-wheels services (home-delivered meal service) and centres for older people. The campaign carried the message "Respect our Elders", and those experiencing maltreatment were directed to adult protection services and a senior helpline (see section 4.4) *(31)*. The campaign included personal stories of maltreatment and support for dealing with abusive situations. The effectiveness of education campaigns interventions remains unknown, since no higher-quality evaluations have been carried out.

**Box 4.3. Protection for whistle-blowers**

Whistle-blowers report malpractice within their organization. Since much maltreatment occurs within institutions and residential care, health professionals may have to decide whether to report maltreatment by a colleague or employer. The use of programmes to encourage reporting of suspected maltreatment (including the use of screening tools) should therefore be accompanied by protocols, policies and legislation that offer protection from reprisals. For instance, in the United Kingdom, the Public Interest Disclosure Act, 1998 protects workers from losing their job, or experiencing any other detriment, as a result of reporting malpractice. Many services also have whistle-blowing policies that set out the standard of behaviour expected of staff and procedures for reporting malpractice.

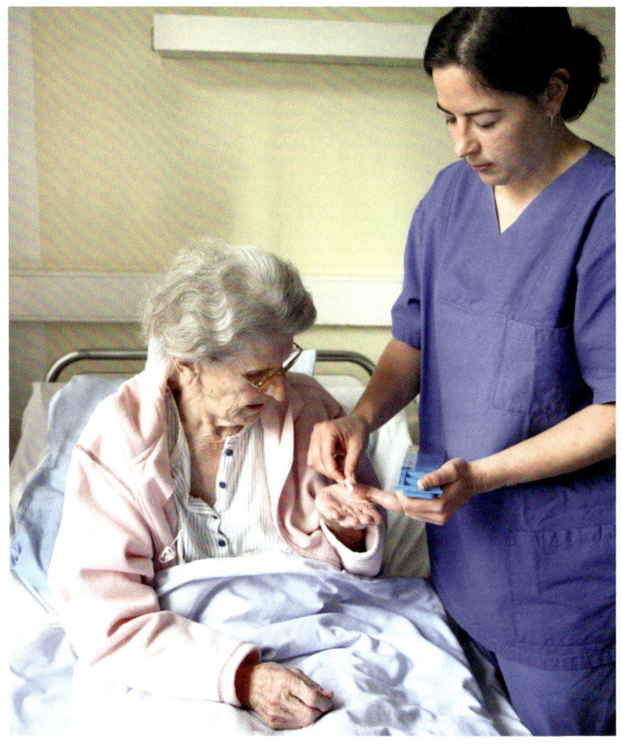

### *4.3.2 Directed at potential maltreaters*

*4.3.2.1 Caregiver education programmes to prevent elder maltreatment*

Among staff members working within nursing and residential care, certain factors appear to play an important role in the development of abusive situations. These include lack of qualifications, a low frustration threshold and caregiver burnout (see Chapter 3). Training programmes have been used to address some of these problems, developing: skills to prevent conflict behaviour with patients; coping mechanisms to deal with difficult patient behaviour; strategies to manage stress; and communication skills (Box 4.4). For instance, in the United States, a maltreatment prevention curriculum was designed for nursing assistants in long-term care facilities. The programme consisted of eight training modules (run over 6–8 hours) that covered: identifying and recognizing maltreatment, risk factors, caregiver stress, cultural and ethnic differences that may lead to conflict with residents, maltreatment of staff by residents and intervention strategies for preventing maltreatment. A variety of teaching methods were used such as role-play scenarios, case discussions or group exercises, sharing experiences of difficult resident behaviour, handouts and a video presentation. The programme established a safe, comfortable environment in which to discuss maltreatment of residents and offered an interactive approach that allowed for open discussion *(32)*. Evaluations of care worker training programmes are generally lacking. Although "weaker" evaluations have reported some positive findings in relation to self-reported abusive behaviour (such as the maltreatment prevention curriculum described above *(32)*), there are no higher-quality evaluations of training programmes from which to draw robust conclusions.

*4.3.2.2 Encouraging positive attitudes among those working with older people*

A further possible risk factor for elder maltreatment is negative attitudes towards older people among care workers or other health workers (see Chapter 3). Some interventions have been undertaken with nursing and medical students to improve attitudes towards older people. These interventions targeted nursing students, nursing assistants and pre-medical students (pre-qualification): those either working or potentially working with older adults. Interventions aimed to encourage more positive attitudes towards older people and older care through educational programmes *(34–36)*, classroom discussion *(37)*, mock (role-playing) geriatric clinics *(37)*, clinical placements *(35,36,38,39)* and intergenerational programmes (see subsection 4.2.3) *(40–42)*, with some interventions combining educational courses and clinical placements. The content of educational programmes and classroom discussion varied, but could include: the ageing process, stereotypes and ageism, expectations about working with older people and the realities of nursing home environments. Higher-quality evaluations of programmes to improve attitudes among nursing and medical students are generally lacking. However, those that exist *(37,40,42)* report a general increase in positive attitudes towards older people in the short term compared with a control group. No evaluation studies have explored subsequent effects on elder maltreatment.

**Box 4.4. Skills in communication for geriatric nurses**

Good communication has an important role to play in the provision of dignified care. The term elderspeak has been used to define a style of communication nurses and other workers use when addressing older people, including simplified communication, louder and slower speech, exaggerated intonation and inappropriate terms of endearment. This style of speech is based on stereotypes that older adults are less competent. However, older people often view this as being patronizing and demeaning, increasing feelings of dependence and reducing the level of perceived control they have over their life. In the United States, a programme was developed for health care workers to raise awareness of elderspeak and the potential negative effects it can have on older adults and to teach good communication skills. Sessions were delivered to nursing assistants using role-play, group discussion, opportunities to practice new skills and videotaped staff–resident interactions. Although there are no high-quality evaluations of the education programme, there was some indication that programme participants became more aware of elderspeak and their own use of this style of communication and fewer incidents of elderspeak occurred following the programme *(33)*.

*4.3.2.3 Informal interventions to support caregivers*

Burnout and stress among caregivers, along with other health and social problems such as depression and lack of social support, can also be risk factors for elder maltreatment among family and other non-paid caregivers such as family or friends (see Chapter 3). Numerous programmes have been developed and tested to support caregivers, promote good mental health and facilitate social interaction. Although the content varies, programmes can provide: information about caring and specific illnesses (such as dementia); skills training to cope with negative emotional states; and opportunities for social interaction with caregivers in similar situations. Numerous formats have been used, of which the main types are education and training programmes *(43,44)*, support groups *(44)*, online information and social support *(45–48)*, respite care *(49–52)* and psychological programmes or therapy *(53–60)*, often including educational components (Box 4.5) *(61-63)*.

## Box 4.5. Examples of psychological and educational programmes within the WHO European Region

Spain

A psychoeducational programme was developed to alleviate stress and burden among caregivers of older people with Alzheimer's disease. Eight sessions were delivered over the course of four months that provided information about the disease, taught strategies for dealing with tension and stress caused by caregiving and taught methods for handling patients' behavioural problems. At a 10-month follow-up, the level of caregiver burden among participants declined versus an increase in a control group. Further, both the well-being and mental health of caregivers improved significantly *(63)*.

Russian Federation

An intervention was developed for the caregivers of older people with dementia. The programme combined education on dementia with training on dealing with problematic behaviour of the people receiving care, such as repeated questioning, clinging or wandering, and was delivered over a five-week period. At a six-month follow-up, compared with a control group, caregiver burden improved significantly, although no differences were found for mental distress or the quality of life of the people receiving care or caregivers *(43)*.

Among the higher-quality evaluations of support interventions, most psychological and educational programmes have been found to reduce the strain and burden of caregivers (Box 4.5) *(43,53,54,62,63)*, although one evaluation *(60)* reported no significant effects. In addition, evaluations of such programmes *(53,55,56,61,62)* report less anxiety or depression associated with participation. There are few higher-quality evaluations for online information and social support programmes. One study in the United States reported no effects on perceived social isolation from a programme that provided a computer network to the caregivers of older people with dementia *(46)*. Lack of higher-quality evaluations is also an issue for respite care; in 2009, a systematic review of respite care *(52)* concluded that, although some evidence supports a positive effect on burden and depression among caregivers, the evidence was limited and weak.

## 4.4 Indicated approaches

### *4.4.1 Involving victims*

#### *4.4.1.1 Adult protective services*

Adult protective services are a part of social services that deals specifically with protecting older people and adults with disabilities from mistreatment or neglect (including self-neglect). This is the model adopted in the United States and used in a few other countries, including Israel. In some instances, separate multidisciplinary response teams have been created alongside adult protective services that work closely with adult protective services and other agencies to respond more efficiently to cases of elder maltreatment or financial exploitation through improved communication and regular meetings. These include elder maltreatment forensic centres *(64,65)*; vulnerable adult or financial abuse specialist teams *(66,67)*; and elder maltreatment prosecution units (Box 4.6) *(68)*. Although most response teams deal specifically with managing and resolving cases of elder maltreatment, some also incorporate a prevention team that raises awareness of elder maltreatment in the community (such as through meals-on-wheels services and pharmacies) and provide tips for prevention. Evaluations of adult protective services are generally lacking. Those available *(64–67,69,70)* are from the United States, focus on professional experiences of adult protective services and are of lower quality. In the United States, there has been some indication that contact with adult protective services can reduce the likelihood of future maltreatment among older victims (by comparing the likelihood of future maltreatment assessed at intake with that assessed at case closure *(70)*). However, since there are no higher-quality evaluations, no confident conclusions may be drawn on the effects of these services.

## Box 4.6. An example of adult protective services in the WHO European Region

In Israel, special units for the preventing and intervening in elder maltreatment have been developed to improve the identification of elder maltreatment and create new modes of intervention. The units have established multidisciplinary teams that include a social worker (coordinator) trained in geriatrics and elder maltreatment, an advising geriatric physician, a lawyer or legal expert and paraprofessionals. Interventions are implemented at an individual level (casework and group therapy) and community level (raising public awareness of the problem). The units provide: legal counselling and representation for older victims, training for social workers and other professionals and evaluation work to establish whether programmes have achieved their goals.

#### *4.4.1.2 Legal, psychological and educational support*

Alongside traditional adult protection services, several interventions have provided additional services for victims, such as legal, psychological and educational support. Those with higher-quality evaluations (from the United States) include the following.

A home-visiting service for victims was combined in some instances with an educational campaign. A police officer and a social worker made the home visit, where discussions took place about current and past maltreatment, legal issues around perpetrating elder maltreatment, procedures for filing a protection order and details of available counselling services *(71,72)*.

A programme involving volunteer advocates provided assistance to victims in using the criminal justice system as well as general social support. Volunteers provided information and help for individuals in pressing charges, help in obtaining a restraining order and assistance in filling out forms and reports *(73)*.

A psychoeducational support group helped older female victims of elder mistreatment. Over the course of eight weeks, the group met and discussed a wide variety of issues relating to maltreatment such as: enhancing self-esteem, dealing with depression, anxiety, stress, coping with loss, strategies for change and further resources for support *(74)*.

Evaluations have reported mixed results. Although the psychoeducational support group did not affect levels of victimization two months later *(74)*, both the home visiting and volunteer advocate programmes reported significantly higher levels of self-reported recurrent maltreatment following the intervention. However, both studies had methodological problems that may have affected the results. Further, interpreting the meaning of the findings is difficult, since the intervention may alter how a person defines (and thus reports) violent behaviour. Nevertheless, a reported increase in abusive behaviour is an important finding and requires further clarification.

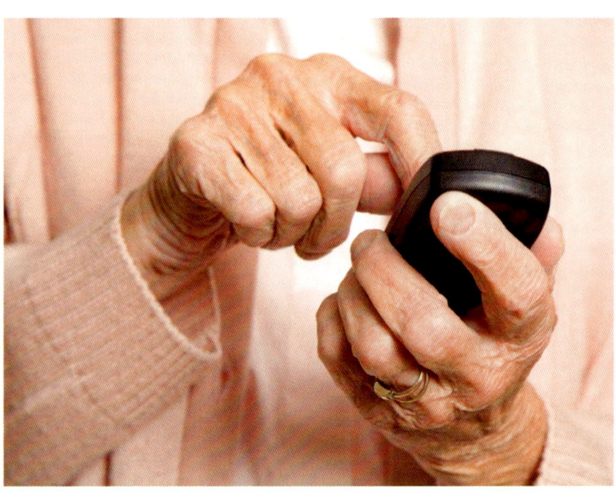

*4.4.1.3 Helplines*

Helplines provide further support for victims of maltreatment. These are usually offered free of charge and provide emotional support as well as information on (and occasionally referrals to) local and national support services. In some cases (such as ALMA France (Box 4.7)), helplines provide follow-up services and ongoing support for callers. There are many examples of helplines across Europe (Box 4.7). Given the often-confidential nature of helplines and the fact that a number of services do not provide follow-up, measuring their effectiveness in preventing subsequent maltreatment can be a challenge. Thus, while analyses of calls to helplines have been evaluated in terms of the types of people calling and the kinds of maltreatment experienced *(75)*, there are no evaluations of specific outcomes relating to elder maltreatment.

**Box 4.7. Examples of elder maltreatment helplines in the WHO European Region**

Germany
Several nongovernmental organization helplines usually operate at the local level. For instance, in Bonn, the helpline Handeln Statt Misshandeln (roughly translates as Action instead of Maltreatment) offers free and confidential advice and help in developing solutions to improve living situations. Handeln Statt Misshandeln also offers home visiting services for those requesting further support (http://www.hsm-bonn.de).

Slovenia
The Centre for Social Work has developed a helpline for older victims of maltreatment. The helpline provides information on support available by the Centre (including emotional support, help contacting police and family support) as well as additional local services (http://www.gov.si/csd/pre_nas_nad_star.htm).

United Kingdom
Action on Elder Abuse runs a free, national helpline for victims of elder maltreatment or people concerned about a friend or relative. The helpline offers information on the nature of elder maltreatment, advice on services available to those affected and emotional support from trained volunteer staff (http://www.elderabuse.org.uk).

France
ALMA France has developed a national network of helpline centres to support and protect older people (and people with disabilities) experiencing maltreatment. The helpline centres are run according to local needs and operated in the first instance by trained volunteers, many of whom are retired with previous experience in health and social care. Unlike most elder maltreatment helplines, professional counsellors follow up initial calls and provide ongoing work (if requested by the caller) to address the maltreatment (http://www.alma-france.org).

#### 4.4.1.4 Emergency shelters

Emergency shelters offer older people temporary, safe accommodation for those who fear remaining in their current living situation. Across Europe, there are many examples of shelters offering support for women who have left an abusive relationship (in particular, for those experiencing intimate partner violence from a current or former partner). These offer counselling and emotional support as well as help in obtaining housing and medical or legal assistance. Although these shelters impose no age restrictions, they are often regarded as shelters for younger women and children. For this reason, some countries (such as Germany) are working with emergency shelters to alter how the public views them and to broaden the targeted age range. In addition, although they are rare, some shelters have been designed specifically for older victims of family maltreatment. These offer emotional support and counselling, legal assistance, health care and help in finding longer-term, safe accommodation (such as the Weinberg Center for Elder Abuse Prevention in Riverdale, New York). Little is known about the effectiveness of emergency shelters in reducing elder maltreatment. There are no evaluations of older people's shelters, and although some studies have explored the effects of women's shelters on quality of life and feelings of safety, there is insufficient evidence to assess their effectiveness on intimate partner revictimization *(76)*.

### 4.4.2 Involving maltreaters

#### 4.4.2.1 Psychological programmes for maltreaters

Psychological programmes have been developed for abusive caregivers with the aim of alleviating or improving the factors contributing to maltreatment such as anger, stress among caregivers and poor coping mechanisms (see Chapter 3). Within such programmes, psychological components (relaxation, stress management or anger management) are often combined with education, covering topics such as a person's illness, the ageing process and elder maltreatment (Box 4.8). Higher-quality evaluations of abusive caregiver programmes are rare but appear to show some promising results. For instance, in Taiwan, evaluations of an educational support group for staff working in nursing homes showed a decrease in staff psychological elder maltreatment behaviour and an increase in knowledge of gerontology compared with a control group. However, there were no changes in staff's perceived levels of work stress *(77)*.

**Box 4.8. An example of a psychological programme for maltreaters**

In the United Kingdom, an education and anger management programme was offered to informal caregivers who had either abused or neglected older people within their care. The programme was provided on a one-to-one basis with a clinical psychologist within two 90-minute sessions (education followed by anger management). The education module provided detailed information about their relatives' illness, information about local services that may provide support (such as respite care) and problems associated with caring for an older person (such as increased social isolation and stress). The anger management component taught about the nature of anger and strategies for dealing with it. Although the programme was evaluated, it did not include a control group for comparison purposes and therefore cannot be considered higher quality. However, significant reductions in factors such as conflict behaviour, strain on caregivers, depression and anxiety were reported following the intervention for the people who either physically abused or neglected a person in their care *(78)*.

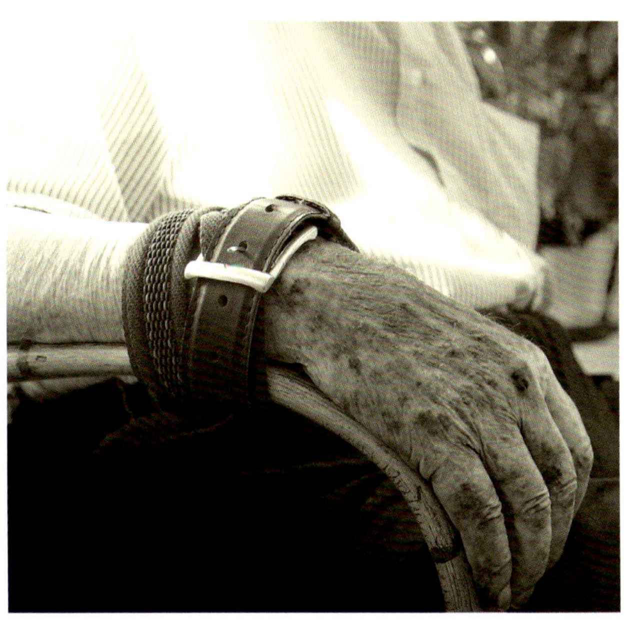

#### 4.4.2.2 Programmes for reducing physical restraints

Within residential and nursing homes and hospitals, nurses and care staff sometimes use physical restraints such as bedrails, belts and chair tables. These restraints are generally used to prevent residents from falling or to control disruptive or distressing behaviour, particularly among people with severe cognitive deficits, such as severe dementia *(79)*. However, there is much debate around their use, since curtailing freedom of movement is considered restrictive, unethical and abusive.

Several interventions have aimed to improve the quality of care provided by professionals by reducing their use of physical restraints. These have included: educational programmes for nurses and care staff (covering information about the nature of common diseases, aggressive patient or resident behaviour and strategies for managing such behaviour); changes in organizational policy that ban the use of restraints; and the use of substitute devices (such as electronic warning devices). A systematic review of such interventions reported five high-quality interventions to prevent and reduce the use of physical restraints in nursing home care. The interventions were all education based and from a variety of countries: the Netherlands, Norway, Sweden and the United States (Box 4.9). The review reported inconsistent findings, with three studies reporting declines in restraint use but one reporting an increase. The study concluded that there was insufficient evidence to support their effectiveness *(80)*. A cluster-randomized controlled trial conducted more recently in 36 nursing homes in Germany provides further support for using education-based interventions. Here, the intervention comprised guidance and a short education session for all nurses within the homes, a one-day workshop and three months of counselling for selected nurses, and brochures for nurses, legal guardians and residents' relatives resulted in a decrease in the use of physical restraints within the nursing homes six months later. Further, no increases were reported in the levels of falls or fractures among older people during the same time period (Meyer G, in preparation).

**Box 4.9. An example of a programme to reduce the use of physical restraints in Sweden**

In Sweden, an education programme was developed to reduce the use of restraints by nursing home staff for older patients with dementia. The programme ran over a six-month period and covered six different themes using videotaped lectures: the symptoms and treatment of people with dementia, delirium among older people, falls and preventing them, the use of physical restraints (including adverse effects and the use of alternative devices), caring for older people with dementia and complications with dementia. Evaluation of the programme reported an improvement in staff attitudes towards the use of physical restraints (becoming less prone to using restraints), and an increase in knowledge of dementia care compared with controls. In addition, the odds of a patient being restrained at follow-up were lower in the intervention group than in the control group *(81)*.

### 4.5 Organizational interventions

A further approach to preventing elder maltreatment focuses on altering or improving professional practice through such methods as developing guidelines and referral protocols and supporting the provision of high-quality care. For instance, in the United States, an integrated system of clinical assessment, service planning and outcome measurement was developed for older people to improve the practices of geriatric mental health care. A toolkit (including but not specific to elder maltreatment) was developed for health professionals that included guidelines on screening, assessment, identification of treatment targets and treatment planning. Feedback on clinical outcomes was also made available to professionals *(82)*.

In the United Kingdom, a care home support team was developed in response to reports of resident maltreatment and aimed to improve standards of care within nursing homes. A multidisciplinary team was created to manage the interface between nursing homes and primary care. Emphasis was placed on supporting care homes by promoting teamwork and professional development, underlining the importance of person-centred care and encouraging staff to examine existing care practices. Work by the care home support team included: workshops offering guidance and facilitated discussion; facilitation of access to e-learning resources; community services and formal training of care home staff; audits; and managerial support *(83)*. Although these programmes have been evaluated, they are of low methodological quality, creating difficulty in drawing any conclusions about their effectiveness.

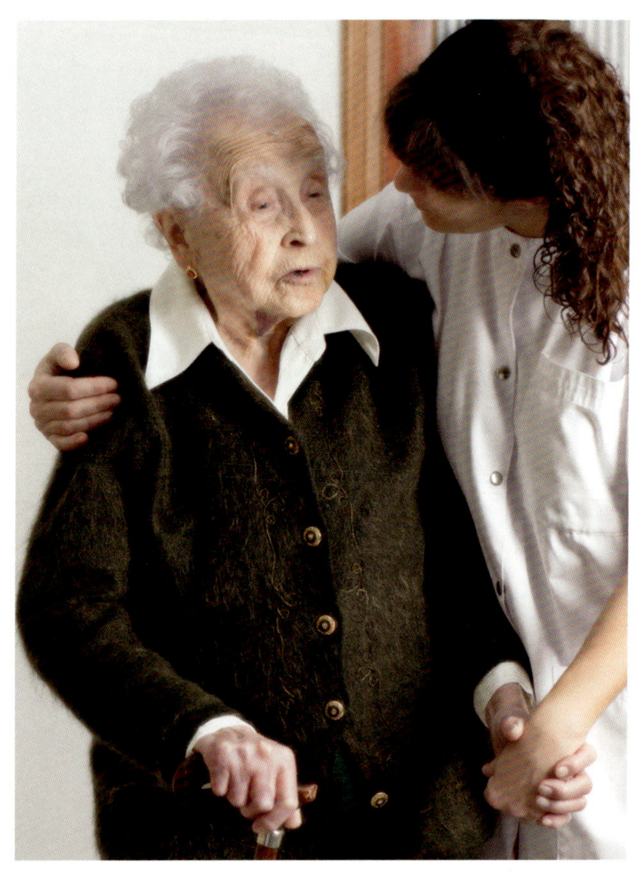

### 4.6 Multi-component interventions

Although most interventions to reduce elder maltreatment have focused on a single strategy, some programmes aim to combine more than one approach to address a range of risk factors for elder maltreatment. For instance, in the United States, a multi-component programme was developed to improve the reporting and management of cases of elder maltreatment, particularly among older people with dementia.

The programme incorporated: educational curricula for professional staff that covered issues of elder maltreatment and dementia as well as effective interventions in dealing with suspected cases; the provision of a screening tool to identify abusive behaviour and potentially abusive situations; a referral and intervention protocol for staff and volunteers in adult protective services; and a handbook for caregivers of people with dementia experiencing strain. The handbook highlighted risks of harm to caregivers and older people with dementia, provided self-assessment instruments in identifying reactions to stress and provided information on where to seek further help and assistance *(84)*. However, there are no higher-quality evaluations of multicomponent programmes.

## 4.7 Discussion

Numerous interventions have been implemented across the European Region that are designed to protect older people from maltreatment, support them in leaving abusive and neglectful situations and improve their quality of care. However, perhaps reflecting a lack of research generally around later life, there are insufficient evaluation studies exploring the effectiveness of interventions on elder maltreatment, both within the European Region and globally. Further, where evaluations exist, they are often of low methodological quality, creating difficulty in quantifying and interpreting the reported effects.

This chapter has included two broad types of intervention: those aiming to reduce or address elder maltreatment and those aiming to improve factors related to elder maltreatment (such as caregiver burden or negative attitudes towards older people). For those that address elder maltreatment specifically, few higher-quality studies are available from which to draw conclusions. Evidence of effectiveness is emerging (evidence from just one higher-quality study) for psychological programmes for maltreaters (subsection 4.4.2.1), which have been associated with a reduction in self-reported abusive behaviour. Further higher-quality evaluations are needed to determine whether these effects can be replicated. There are mixed findings for the effectiveness of: professional awareness and education courses (subsection 4.2.2; mixed results); legal, psychological and educational support programmes (subsection 4.4.1.2; mixed results); and restraint reduction programmes (subsection 4.4.2.2; mixed results). However, importantly, several evaluations have reported an increase in maltreatment following the intervention (such as home visiting programmes, volunteer advocates (subsection 4.4.1.2) and restraint reduction programmes (subsection 4.4.2.2)). Although interpreting what these results represent is difficult (such as an actual increase in abusive behaviour, changes in understanding of what constitutes maltreatment or methodological flaws in research design), it seems clear that further research is needed to clarify any potentially harmful effects of intervention on older victims of maltreatment.

No higher-quality evaluations include elder maltreatment outcomes for: public information campaigns; screening; education campaigns for potential victims of maltreatment; caregiver education programmes to prevent elder maltreatment; adult protective services; helplines; emergency shelters; organizational interventions; or multicomponent interventions despite the frequent use of some of these programmes (such as helplines) throughout the European Region and else. For interventions that aim to reduce factors relating to maltreatment, there is promising evidence of effectiveness (evidence from several evaluation studies) for: school-based intergenerational programmes (subsection 4.2.3), programmes that encourage positive attitudes among those working with older people (subsection 4.3.2.2) and informal caregiver support programmes (subsection 4.3.2.3). All three interventions have been associated with positive changes at least in the short term (such as improved attitudes towards ageing and older people and decreased caregiver stress, burden and depression). Importantly, however, very little known is still about whether these changes affect levels of current or future elder maltreatment perpetration. This is further compounded by a lack of longer-term evaluation studies, meaning that the sustainability of even the reported effects is unknown.

### Key messages

Wherever possible, programmes should be implemented using an evaluative framework that includes elder maltreatment outcomes, longer-term follow-up and cost–effectiveness.

Further research is needed to clarify the apparent increases in maltreatment reported following some interventions. This should help explain why reported increases might occur and how such results should be interpreted.

Further research is also needed on the costs associated with implementing elder maltreatment interventions.

Based on the evaluation studies included in this chapter, very little can be concluded about which interventions may be most effective in reducing or preventing elder maltreatment. Further, there is no information on the costs of implementing programmes. However, there are numerous examples of interventions that have been implemented across the European Region. Although the evidence on which they are based is largely absent, their development at least suggests that governments and organizations have begun to recognize this social problem and want to address it.

Although rigorous evaluation may present challenges for some types of programme (such as public information campaigns), the development of high-quality evidence is essential for informing practitioners and policy-makers of the most effective (and cost-effective) interventions. With little evidence on what can prevent elder maltreatment, existing and any new programmes must use good evaluative frameworks that not only examine improvements in practices, knowledge and reporting but also directly measure the effects on elder maltreatment.

## 4.8 References


1. Ploeg J et al. A systematic review of interventions for elder abuse. *Journal of Elder Abuse and Neglect*, 2009, 21:187–210.

2. Pillemer K et al. Interventions to prevent elder mistreatment. In: Doll LS et al., eds. *Handbook of injury and violence prevention*. New York, Springer, 2008.

3. *Preventing violence through the development of safe, stable and nurturing relationships between children and their parents and caregivers.* Geneva, World Health Organization, 2009 (http://www.who.int/violence_injury_prevention/violence/4th_milestones_meeting/publications/en/index.html, accessed 9 May 2011).

4. *Preventing violence by developing life skills in children and adolescents*. Geneva, World Health Organization, 2009 (http://www.who.int/violence_injury_prevention/violence/4th_milestones_meeting/publications/en/index.html, accessed 9 May 2011).

5. *HSE elder abuse services, 2009*. London, Health Service Executive, 2009 (http://www.hse.ie/eng/services/Publications/services/Older/openyoureyes.pdf, accessed 9 May 2011).

6. Day MR, Bantry-White E, Glavin P. Protection of vulnerable adults: an interdisciplinary workshop. *Community Practitioner*, 2010, 83:29–32.

7. McGarry J, Simpson C. Nursing students and elder abuse: developing a learning resource. *Nursing Older People*, 2009, 19:27–30.

8. Désy PM, Prohaska TR. The Geriatric Emergency Nursing Education (GENE) course: an evaluation. *Journal of Emergency Nursing*, 2008, 34:396–402.

9. Richardson B, Kitchen G, Livingstone G. The effect of education on knowledge and management of elder abuse: a randomized controlled trial. *Age and Ageing*, 2002, 31:335–341.

10. Laditka SB et al. There's no place like home: evaluating family medicine residents' training in home care. *Home Health Care Services Quarterly*, 2002, 21:1–17.

11. Jogerst GJ, Ely JW. Home visit program for teaching elder abuse evaluations. *Family Medicine*, 1997, 29:634–639.

12. Smith MK et al. Twelve important minutes: introducing enhanced online materials about elder abuse to nursing assistants. *Journal of Continuing Education in Nursing*, 2010, 41:281–288.

13. Krug E et al., eds. *World report on violence and health*. Geneva, World Health Organization, 2002 (http://www.who.int/violence_injury_prevention/violence/world_report/en, accessed 9 May 2011).

14. Aday RH, McDuffie W, Rice Sims C. Impact of an intergenerational program on black adolescents' attitudes toward the elderly. *Educational Gerontology*, 1993, 19:663–673.

15. Cummings SM, Williams MM, Ellis RA. Impact of an intergenerational program on 4th graders' attitudes towards elders and school behaviours. *Journal of Human Behaviour in the Social Environment*, 2003, 8:43–61.

16. Dellman-Jenkins M et al. Intergenerational sharing seminars: their impact on young adult college students and senior guest students. *Educational Gerontology*, 1994, 20:579–588.

17. Kassab C, Cance L. An assessment of the effectiveness of an intergenerational program for youth. *Psychological Reports*, 1999, 84:198–200.

18. Chapman NJ, Neal MB. The effects of intergenerational experiences on adolescents and older adults. *The Gerontologist*, 1990, 30:825–832.

19. Kaplan MS. Intergenerational programs in schools: consideration of form and function. *International Review of Education*, 2002, 48:30–334.

20. Couper DP, Sheehan NW, Thomas EL. Attitude toward old people: the impact of an intergeneration program. *Educational Gerontology*, 1991, 17:41–53.

21. Hannon PO, Gueldner SH. The impact of short-term quality intergenerational contact on children's attitudes towards older adults. *Journal of Intergenerational Relationships*, 2007, 5(4):59–76.

22. Dellmann-Jenkins M, Lambert D, Fruit D. Fostering preschoolers' prosocial behaviours toward the elderly: the effect of an intergenerational program. *Educational Gerontology*, 1991, 17:21–32.

23. Aday RH et al. Changing children's attitudes toward the elderly: the longitudinal effects of an intergenerational partners program. *Journal of Research in Childhood Education*, 1996, 10:143–150.

24. Aday RH, Sims CR, Evans E. Youth's attitudes toward the elderly: the impact of intergenerational partners. *Journal of Applied Gerontology*, 1991, 19:372–384.

25. Reis M, Nahmiash D. Validation of the Indicators of Abuse (IOA) screen. *The Gerontologist*, 1998, 38:471–480.

26. Yaffe MJ et al. Development and validation of a tool to improve physician identification of elder abuse: the Elder Abuse Suspicion Index (EASI)©. *Journal of Elder Abuse and Neglect*, 2008, 20:276–300.

27. Cohen M et al. Development of a screening tool for identifying elderly people at risk of abuse by their caregivers. *Journal of Ageing and Health*, 2006, 18:660–685.

28. Wang JJ, Tseng HF, Chen KM. Development and testing of screening indicators for psychological abuse of older people. *Archives of Psychiatric Nursing*, 2007, 21:40–47.

29. Acierno R et al. Assessing elder victimization. *Social Psychiatry and Psychiatric Epidemiology*, 2003, 38:644–653.

30. Beach SR et al. Using audio computer-assisted self-interviewing and interactive voice response to measure elder mistreatment in older adults: feasibility and effects on prevalence estimates. *Journal of Official Statistics*, 2010, 26:507–533.

31. *Center for Crime Victim Services launches public education campaign*. Waterbury, Vermont Center for Crime Victim Services (http://www.ccvs.state.vt.us/pub_ed/launch.html, accessed 9 May 2011).

32. Pillemer K, Hudson B. A model abuse prevention program for nursing assistants. *The Gerontologist*, 1993, 33:128–131.

33. Williams K, Kemper S, Hummert L. Enhancing communication with older adults: overcoming elderspeak. *Journal of Gerontological Nursing*, 2004, 30(10):17–25.

34. Williams B, Anderson MC, Day R. Undergraduate nursing students' knowledge of and attitudes towards aging: comparison of context-based learning and a traditional program. *Journal of Nursing Education*, 2007, 46:115–120.

35. Rogan F, Wyllie A. Engaging undergraduate nursing students in the care of elderly residents in Australian nursing homes. *Nurse Education in Practice*, 2003, 3:95–103.

36. Fox SD, Wold JE. Baccalaureate student gerontological nursing experiences: raising consciousness levels and affecting attitudes. *Journal of Nursing Education*, 1996, 35:348–355.

37. Brown DS et al. Improvement in attitudes toward the elderly following traditional and geriatric mock clinics for physical therapy students. *Physical Therapy*, 1992, 72:251–257.

38. Sheffler SJ. Do clinical experiences affect nursing students' attitudes toward the elderly? *Journal of Nursing Education*, 1995, 34:312–316.

39. Hartley C, Bentz PM, Ellis JR. The effect of early nursing home placement on student attitudes toward the elderly. *Journal of Nursing Education*, 1995, 34:128–130.

40. Gonzales E, Morrow-Howell N, Gilbert P. Changing medical students' attitudes toward older adults. *Gerontology and Geriatrics Education*, 2010, 31:220–234.

41. Butler FR, Baghi H. Using the Internet to facilitate positive attitudes of college students toward aging and working with older adults. *Journal of Intergenerational Relationships*, 2008, 6:175–189.

42. Dorfman LT et al. Incorporating intergenerational service-learning into an introductory gerontology course. *Journal of Gerontological Social Work*, 2003, 39:219–240.

43. Gavrilova SI et al. Helping carers to care – the 10/66 dementia research group's randomized control trial of a caregiver intervention in Russia. *International Journal of Geriatric Psychiatry*, 2009, 24:347–354.

44. Donorfio LKM, Vetter R, Vracevic M. Effects of three caregiver interventions: support, educational literature and creative movement. *Journal of Women and Aging*, 2010, 22:61–75.

45. Torp S et al. A pilot study of how information and communication technology may contribute to health promotion among elderly spousal carers in Norway.

*Health and Social Care in the Community*, 2008, 16:75–85.

46. Brennan PF, Moore SM, Smyth KA. The effects of a special computer network on caregivers of persons with Alzheimer's disease. *Nursing Research*, 1995, 44:166–172.

47. Dow B et al. Rural carers online: a feasibility study. *Australian Journal of Rural Health*, 2008, 16:221–225.

48. Glueckauf RL, Loomis JS. Alzheimer's caregiver support online: lessons learned, initial findings and future directions. *NeuroRehabilitation*, 2003, 18:135–146.

49. Perry J, Bontinen K. Evaluation of a weekend respite program for persons with Alzheimer disease. *Canadian Journal of Nursing Research*, 2001, 33:81–95.

50. Gaugler JE, Zarit SH. The effectiveness of adult day services for disabled older people. *Journal of Aging and Social Policy*, 2001, 12(2):23–47.

51. Shaw C et al. Systematic review of respite care in the frail elderly. *Health Technology Assessment*, 2009, 13(20):1–224.

52. Mason A et al. The effectiveness and cost-effectiveness of respite for caregivers of frail older people. *Journal of the American Geriatrics Society*, 2007, 55:290–299.

53. López J, Crespo M. Analysis of the efficacy of a psychotherapeutic program to improve the emotional status of caregivers of elderly dependent relatives. *Aging and Mental Health*, 2008, 12:451–461.

54. Andrén S, Elmståhl S. Psychosocial intervention for family caregivers of people with dementia reduces caregiver's burden: development and effect after 6 and 12 months. *Nordic College of Caring Sciences*, 2008, 22:98–109.

55. Coon DW et al. Anger and depression management: psychoeducational skill training interventions for women caregivers of a relative with dementia. *The Gerontologist*, 2003, 43:678–689.

56. Eisdorfer C et al. The effect of a family therapy and technology-based intervention on caregiver depression. *The Gerontologist*, 2003, 43:521–531.

57. Huynh-Hohnbaum AT et al. Evaluating a multicomponent caregiver intervention. *Home Health Care Services Quarterly*, 2008, 27:299–324.

58. Gallagher-Thompson D, Coon DW. Evidence-based psychological treatment for distress in family caregivers of older adults. *Psychology and Aging*, 2007, 22:37–51.

59. Tompkins SA, Bell PA. Examination of a psychoeducational intervention and a respite grant in relieving psychosocial stressors associated with being an Alzheimer's caregiver. *Journal of Gerontological Social Work*, 2009, 52:89–104.

60. Scogin F et al. Training for abusive caregivers: an unconventional approach to an intervention dilemma. *Journal of Elder Abuse and Neglect*, 1990, 1(4):73–86.

61. Belle SH et al. Enhancing the quality of life of dementia caregivers from different ethnic or racial groups. *Annals of Internal Medicine*, 2006, 145:727–738.

62. Elliot A, Burgio LD, DeCoster J. Enhancing caregiver health: findings from the resources for enhancing Alzheimer's caregiver health II intervention. *Journal of the American Geriatrics Society*, 2010, 58:30–37.

63. Martín-Carrasco M et al. Effectiveness of a psychoeducational intervention program in the reduction of caregiver burden in Alzheimer's disease patients' caregivers. *International Journal of Geriatric Psychiatry*, 2009, 24:489–499.

64. Navarro AE et al. Do we really need another meeting? Lessons from the Los Angeles County Elder Abuse Forensic Center. *The Gerontologist*, 2010, 50:702–711.

65. Wiglesworth A et al. Findings from an Elder Abuse Forensic Center. *The Gerontologist*, 2006, 46:277–283.

66. Malks B, Schmidt CM, Austin MJ. Elder abuse prevention: a case study of the Santa Clara County Financial Abuse Specialist Team (FAST) program. *Journal of Gerontological Social Work*, 2002, 39(3): 23–40.

67. Mosqueda L et al. Advancing the field of elder mistreatment: a new model for integration of social and medical services. *The Gerontologist*, 44:703–708.

68. Velasco JG. Ventura County District Attorney's Senior Crime Prevention program. *Journal of Elder Abuse and Neglect*, 2000, 12:10–106.

69. Dauenhauer JA, Mayer KC, Mason A. Evaluation of adult protective services: perspectives of community

professionals. *Journal of Elder Abuse and Neglect*, 2007, 19(3/4):41–57.

70. Neale AV et al. The Illinois elder abuse system: program description and administrative findings. *The Gerontologist*, 1996, 36:502–511.

71. Davis RC, Medina-Ariza J. *Results from an elder abuse prevention experiment in New York City*. National Institute of Justice: research in brief. New York, National Institute of Justice, 2001 (http://www.ncjrs.gov/pdffiles1/nij/188675.pdf, accessed 9 May 2011).

72. Davis RC, Medina J, Avitabile N. *Reducing repeat incidents of elder abuse: results of a randomized experiment*. New York, Victims Research Service, 2000 (http://www.ncjrs.gov/pdffiles1/nij/grants/189086.pdf, accessed 9 May 2011).

73. Filinson R. An evaluation of a program of volunteer advocates for elder abuse victims. *Journal of Elder Abuse and Neglect*, 1993, 5:77–94.

74. Brownell P, Heiser D. Psycho-educational support groups for older women victims of family mistreatment: a pilot study. *Journal of Gerontological Social Work*, 2006, 46(3–4):145–160.

75. Action on Elder Abuse. *Hidden voices: older people's experience of abuse. An analysis of calls to the Action on Elder Abuse helpline.* London, Help the Aged, 2004.

76. *Reducing violence through victim identification, care and support programmes*. Geneva, World Health Organization, 2008 (http://www.who.int/violence_injury_prevention/violence/4th_milestones_meeting/publications/en/index.html, accessed 9 May 2011).

77. Hsieh H et al. Educational support group in changing caregivers' psychological elder abuse behaviour toward caring for institutionalized elders. *Advances in Health and Science Education*, 2009, 14:377–386.

78. Campbell Reay AM, Browne KD. The effectiveness of psychological interventions with individuals who physically abuse or neglect their elderly dependents. *Journal of Interpersonal Violence*, 2002, 17:416–431.

79. Bredhauer D et al. Factors relating to the use of physical restraint in psychogeriatric care: a paradigm for elder abuse. *Zeitschrift fur Gerontologie und Geriatrie*, 2005, 38:10–18.

80. Möhler R et al. Interventions for preventing and reducing the use of physical restraints in long-term geriatric care. *Cochrane Database of Systematic Reviews* 2011, (2):CD007546.

81. Pellfolk THE et al. Effects of a restraint minimization program on staff knowledge, attitudes and practice: a cluster randomized trial. *Journal of the American Geriatrics Society*, 2010, 58:62–69.

82. Bartels SJ et al. Improving mental health assessment and service planning practices for older adults: a controlled comparison study. *Mental Health Services Research*, 2005, 7:213–223.

83. Lawrence V, Banerjee S. Improving care in care homes: a qualitative evaluation of the Croydon care home support team. *Aging and Mental Health*, 2010, 14:416–424.

84. Anetzberger GJ et al. A model intervention for elder abuse and dementia. *The Gerontologist*, 2000, 40:492–497.

# 5. Policy and programming

## 5.1 Findings of the report

Elder maltreatment is a problem endemic in all countries in the European Region.

### *5.1.1 Why elder maltreatment matters in the European Region*

There are 8300 older people dying from homicide each year in the European Region, and an estimated 30% of these are from elder maltreatment. Prevalence studies suggest that, every year, 2.7% of older people suffer from elder maltreatment in the form of physical abuse, 0.7% sexual abuse, 19.4% mental abuse and 3.8% financial abuse. Applying these estimates to the European Region implies that at least 4 million people experience elder maltreatment as physical abuse in any one year. For financial abuse, this is estimated at almost 6 million and for mental abuse at almost 29 million. Victims of maltreatment may concurrently experience more than one type of abuse or neglect. There are grave long-term consequences that affect older people's health and mental well-being and lead to increase demands on services, social isolation and premature death. The effects of the different types of maltreatment need to be better understood. In addition to the additional burden posed to the health sector and the demands on social and criminal justice services are the high social costs of the effects on the people and families affected by maltreatment. Longitudinal studies are needed to better understand the long-term health and social consequences of elder maltreatment.

Elder maltreatment is increasingly being recognized as a health and social problem *(1–3)*. Within the Region, concern is growing about elder maltreatment, especially in countries with an ageing population. A recent survey of health ministry focal people for violence prevention with 40 respondent countries from across the Region confirmed this interest (Fig. 5.1) (Annex 3 has the questionnaire, and Annex 1 provides details on the process). Elder maltreatment is perceived as a very great problem in 3% of countries, as a great problem in 8% of countries and as a moderate problem in 38% of countries. In 38% of the countries it is perceived as a slight problem and no problem at all in 13%. The vast majority of focal people were interested in receiving more information on elder maltreatment. This is in accordance with findings from a recent Eurobarometer survey of residents in EU countries *(4)*. This reported that nearly half of those surveyed consider poor treatment, neglect and even abuse of older people to be fairly or very widespread in their country. More than two thirds (67%) felt that older people are financially exploited and receive inadequate care, and most felt that this vulnerable group is at risk of mental and physical abuse. One third of the respondents perceived the perpetrators to be staff in a care home or a home care worker, and nearly one quarter of the respondents said that older people's children are the perpetrators.

### *5.1.2 Older people are vulnerable to maltreatment*

In old age, people may develop ill health, become frail and be unable to live independently, thus increasing their dependence on other people. This makes them potentially more vulnerable to maltreatment in all settings, and this is particularly true of those who are older and more disabled and dependent. The trust that older people put in other people to look after them should not be broken. Given the growing population of older people and the existing scale of the problem, preventing elder maltreatment and protecting older people should be a key policy priority, as this report outlines.

Societal attitudes of ageism and negative attitudes towards older people and stereotyping of the older people devalue and marginalize many older people. This can negatively influence self-esteem, worsen social exclusion, reduce a sense of social control and worsen the well-being and quality of life of older people. Elder maltreatment is one of the most hidden forms of violence and neglect in the European Region and should be a key priority for government responses. It is an important manifestation of interpersonal violence occurring in families, an intergenerational concern as well as a public health, justice and human rights issue. Similar to children, much is to be gained by ensuring that older people have a right to live in safe environments *(5)*. Member States need to ensure that older people can live with dignity, integrity and independence and without maltreatment.

### *5.1.3 A time of rapid change and increasing inequality in the European Region*

Rising life expectancy and low birth rates imply profound change in the current balance between generations. Moreover, it is feared that, in many countries, the older generation is becoming too severe a burden on the younger generation, and this could result in increased tensions between the generations and rising inequality *(6,7)*. These demographic shifts heighten the relevance of socioeconomic factors affecting older people. In particular, the physical, mental and financial vulnerability and dependence of many older people continues to heighten concern about the risk of inequality and maltreatment that older people may face.

The economic downturn has further impoverished many older people. This has been superimposed on the

**Fig. 5.1. A questionnaire survey – country-specific results**

| Countries | Is elder maltreatment a problem? | Is elder maltreatment perceived as a problem? | Is there a national policy on elder maltreatment? | Are there estimates of the proportion of homicides among older people caused by elder maltreatment? | Is there interest in having more information on elder maltreatment? | Is there a research institute or university concerned with elder maltreatment? |
|---|---|---|---|---|---|---|
| Serbia | It is a big problem | It is a big problem | Yes | Yes | Yes | No |
| Austria | It is a big problem | It is a big problem | Yes, in some areas | I don't know | Yes | Yes |
| Israel | It is a big problem | It is a moderate problem | Yes | I don't know | Yes | Yes |
| The former Yugoslav Republic of Macedonia | It is a big problem | It is a moderate problem | No | Yes | Yes | No |
| Portugal | It is a big problem | It is a moderate problem | Yes, in some areas | Yes | Yes | Yes |
| Slovakia | It is a big problem | It is a slight problem | No | No | Yes | Yes |
| Cyprus | It is a moderate problem | It is a very big problem | Yes | No | Yes | Yes |
| Netherlands | It is a moderate problem | It is a big problem | Yes | I don't know | Yes | Yes |
| Bosnia and Herzegovina[a] | It is a moderate problem | It is a moderate problem | Yes | No answer | Yes | No answer |
| Montenegro | It is a moderate problem | It is a moderate problem | Yes | Yes | Yes | Yes |
| Slovenia | It is a moderate problem | It is a moderate problem | Yes | No | Yes | Yes |
| United Kingdom | It is a moderate problem | It is a moderate problem | Yes | No | Yes | No |
| Czech Republic | It is a moderate problem | It is a moderate problem | No | I don't know | Yes | Yes |
| Finland | It is a moderate problem | It is a moderate problem | No | I don't know | Yes | Yes |
| Greece | It is a moderate problem | It is a moderate problem | No | I don't know | Yes | No |
| Iceland | It is a moderate problem | It is a moderate problem | No | No | Yes | Yes |
| Romania | It is a moderate problem | It is a moderate problem | No | I don't know | Yes | No |
| Belgium | It is a moderate problem | It is a moderate problem | Yes, in some areas | No | Yes | Yes |
| Russian Federation | It is a moderate problem | It is a moderate problem | Yes, in some areas | I don't know | Yes | No |
| Bulgaria | It is a moderate problem | It is a slight problem | No | No | Yes | Yes |
| Croatia | It is a moderate problem | It is a slight problem | No | No | Yes | Yes |
| Lithuania | It is a moderate problem | It is a slight problem | No | No | Yes | No |
| Latvia | It is a moderate problem | It is a slight problem | No | No | Yes | No |
| Norway | It is a moderate problem | It is a slight problem | No | No | Yes | Yes |
| Spain | It is a moderate problem | It is a slight problem | No | I don't know | Yes | No |
| Malta | It is a moderate problem | It is a slight problem | No | No | Yes | Yes |
| Switzerland | It is a moderate problem | It is a slight problem | Yes, in some areas | No | Yes | Yes |
| Tajikistan | It is a moderate problem | It is not a problem at all | No | No answer | Yes | No |
| Germany | It is a slight problem | It is a slight problem | Yes | I don't know | Yes | Yes |
| Estonia | It is a slight problem | It is a slight problem | No | No answer | No answer | No answer |
| Ireland | It is a slight problem | It is a slight problem | Yes | No | Yes | Yes |
| Albania | It is a slight problem | It is a slight problem | No | No | Yes | Yes |
| Azerbaijan | It is a slight problem | It is a slight problem | No | No | Yes | No |
| San Marino | It is a slight problem | It is a slight problem | Yes, in some areas | No | Yes | No |
| Denmark | It is a slight problem | It is not a problem at all | No | Yes | No | No |
| Italy | It is a slight problem | It is not a problem at all | No | I don't know | Yes | No |
| Uzbekistan | It is not a problem at all | It is not a problem at all | No | Yes | Yes | No |
| Armenia | It is not a problem at all | It is not a problem at all | Yes, in some areas | No | Yes | No |
| Andorra | No answer | No answer | No answer | No answer | No answer | No answer |

Legends: It is a very big problem; It is a big problem; It is a moderate problem; It is a slight problem; It is not a problem at all; Yes; Yes, in some areas; No; I don't know; No answer

[a]Only the Republic of Srpska.

*Source*: results of a WHO questionnaire survey.

socioeconomic and political transition that many countries have undergone with the loss of social support networks and may have led to increased social strain, which has adversely affected older people with lower incomes, making them more susceptible to violence *(8)*. Where there are no welfare support structures, older people depend on the voluntary commitment of their families *(9)*. The transition into a caregiving situation can be highly stressful for family members, especially when the conditions requiring care are long term and progressive, which applies to many illnesses in later life *(10)*. This increasing stress on family members caring for older adults may result in rising levels of maltreatment, and this may affect disproportionately affect families with fewer socioeconomic resources. The high prevalence of elder maltreatment highlighted in this report and its reflection in the concerns of policy-makers (see subsection 5.1.2) clearly indicate that elder maltreatment is a public health and societal problem that needs to be addressed and is a matter of social justice.

### *5.1.4 Elder maltreatment should be prevented*

This report presents the available evidence on the burden and risk factors and emphasizes that older people are often potentially vulnerable to maltreatment. The causes of their maltreatment are structural, linked to social determinants and intergenerational factors; they are also often related to alcohol or drug misuse and to inadequate social support networks. In accordance with the public health framework proposed by the *World report on violence and health (11)*, elder maltreatment should be preventable. What is striking, as summarized in Chapter 4, is the lack of evidence-informed, population-based and theory-founded programmes. Instead, individual needs-based responses have been proposed. Although these have been effective in focusing greater attention on the problem, little reliable information is available that can inform policy-makers of the benefits of programmes relative to the costs. This is similar to the response to domestic violence and child maltreatment, which has focused until recently on protection rather than prevention. Outcome-based research on preventing elder maltreatment is urgently needed *(12)*.

## 5.2 The way forward

### *5.2.1 Need for better data*

One challenge facing the response to elder maltreatment is the need for uniform definitions between agencies. Good information systems are needed to support policy-makers, practitioners and advocates in shaping and guiding their choices and in evaluating and monitoring programmes and policy *(13,14)*. As highlighted in this report, there is little routine information on this at either the local or national level. Many countries in the European Region collect and collate data on the maltreatment of older people in different ways. Problems in definitions and methods also result in difficulty in assessing the scale of the problem and understanding risk factors, which then create difficulty in comparing data from various countries. In addition, elder maltreatment is a "hidden" issue that usually occurs in the privacy of the home and is viewed as a family affair; further, there may be limited access to institutional settings. Mortality data are incompletely coded, and data from health and other statutory services underrepresent the scale of the problem. For example, for every case reported, an estimated 20 are not known about *(15)*. Few countries are taking a systematic approach to improve data (Box 5.1). For example, in the United States, there is current emphasis on developing uniform definitions and surveillance systems to allow for multiagency data collection and sharing *(16)*. Much of the data in the European Region are based on surveys from selected countries (see section 2.4), and few are from the eastern part of the Region. There are plans to undertake a survey in the former Yugoslav Republic of Macedonia (Box 5.2).

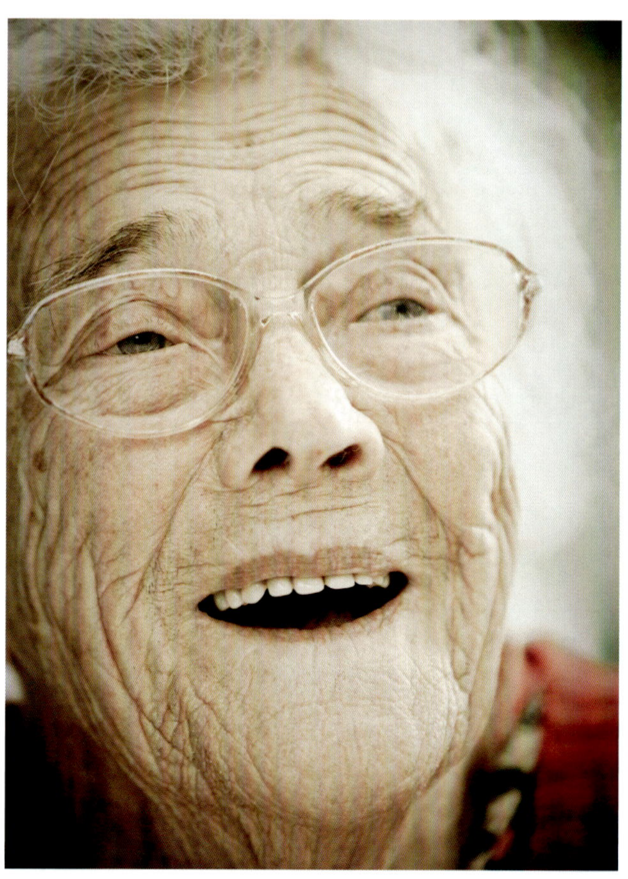

### *5.2.2 Ensuring better governance for the care of older people*

The health and social welfare sectors play a key role in ensuring high standards of care and treatment. This applies across all settings – family homes, nursing or care homes and hospitals. Many countries already have a substantial policy and legislative framework that can be used to counter elder maltreatment. In some circumstances, an act or omission is a criminal offence; others violate professional codes or service standards or breach human rights.

### Box 5.1. Local data – examples from the United Kingdom

Two examples of data that are collected systematically in most areas are from England and Wales. First, adult safeguarding boards produce annual reports, which are a valuable potential source of data on the mistreatment of vulnerable people. Second, in 2010 the NHS National Information Centre for Health and Social Care set up a data collection system to draw together information on referrals to local councils about the abuse and neglect of vulnerable adults, including people living in care homes or being treated in hospitals. The first results of this will be published in 2011. It is anticipated that this will be the best source of data so far on the reported abuse and neglect of older people (and other adults) in care homes or hospitals (and all other settings) in England and Wales.

Local interest groups and older people's organizations can use such data to promote the health and well-being of older people. For example, in Wales, a pressure group called A Dignified Revolution – comprising relatives and older people themselves – has passionately advocated the need to improve the quality of care for older people in hospitals and all other settings. The group uses Internet communication to monitor examples of poor practice and to pass on details of positive developments. It engages with policy-makers, particularly at the level of the Welsh Assembly Government.

*Source:* Manthorpe *(17)*.

Regulatory bodies for institutions in many countries have a system of regulation, inspection and quality assurance that includes protecting older people from maltreatment. Many professionals working with older people have some form of professional regulatory body, which should play a role in protecting older people from mistreatment. These bodies should ensure high standards of training and care and ensure the accountability of health and care professionals concerning complaints by older people and their families. These standards need to be uniformly high, especially given the professional and non-professional staff mobility in the European Region and ensuring that older people have confidence in their health and care professionals. Many countries have no common system or registry of care assistants working in care homes or people supporting older people in their own homes. There is substantial migration of care workers within the Region, and standards of care need to be maintained both formally and informally. Much informal care is provided in people's own homes, and this may represent an opportunity for improving standards (Box 5.3).

### Box 5.2. National response to elder maltreatment in the former Yugoslav Republic of Macedonia

After independence, the former Yugoslav Republic of Macedonia has gone through a period of transition, which has affected the health care system and contributed to the loss of social networks in common with most countries in south-eastern Europe. Unemployment has risen to 32% *(18)*. This means that older people who have pensions very often have the only income in the family, making younger generations dependent on them. Increased physical and mental dependence on family members often makes older people more susceptible to maltreatment. People aged 60 years and older represent 11.6% of the population, and this is expected to increase. Elder maltreatment has only received attention recently.

The national report on violence and health *(19)* emphasized elder maltreatment as a public health concern. The national strategy for combating domestic violence for 2008–2012 addressed some of the recommendations made. So far, the focus has been on intimate partner violence among older people by developing protocols for the health, social, educational, police and nongovernmental organization sectors. The only data on elder maltreatment are based on reports of maltreatment to agencies for domestic violence *(20)*. Whereas 4% of reported cases of intimate partner violence are among older people, this is higher (17%) in calls received by the national helpline for victims of domestic violence in 2010. Of the calls by people older than 65 years, 35% reported suffering maltreatment from their children or grandchildren. Civil society has responded to the problem by offering increased peer support for informal measures, and several nongovernmental organizations are very active in improving the quality of life of older people through life-long learning and providing support for those in need. Further educational programmes for primary health care workers focus on positive attitudes towards older people, training in case detection and prevention through early treatment of depression and detection of Alzheimer's disease among groups at higher risk.

The following steps are being planned:

- a national prevalence survey to identify the scale, risks and consequences;
- developing a national strategy on preventing elder maltreatment;
- improving access to services that will support victims such as telephone helplines, emergency care, safe-houses, health and legal action and counselling; and
- improving case detection and referral for protection.

**Box 5.3. Civil society response to caring for older people in Italy**

Italy's life expectancy is among the highest in the European Region in both sexes, and the population is rapidly ageing similar to other countries in the Region. Italy has the highest old-age dependency index in the European Region. Of the almost 12 million people older than 65 years, 3% are cared for in nursing or residential homes. This is low compared with other EU countries. The remainder (11.5 million) live at home, and this may be in multigenerational families, although this lifestyle is now declining. There is a north–south divide, and 73% of older people in residential homes are in the north. About 60% of the residential homes are privately run, putting a financial strain on families that do not qualify for state assistance (62%). Most older people therefore receive care at home. To reduce the burden on the family, many families have chosen to employ care workers to look after older people. A decline by half in the percentage of people older than 85 years in residential care has been attributed primarily to the employment of home care workers from outside Italy, mainly from eastern Europe. There may be an estimated 700 000 legally registered care workers in homes in Italy, equivalent to 50% of the total number of registered workers in private home care, and in 75% of cases they live with people older than 75 years old who need care. Illegal care workers need to be added to this figure. This is more affordable than nursing homes. There may be opportunities for training such care workers to promote their caregiving skills and to better safeguard older people in their care.

*Sources*: Mestheneos et al. *(21)*; Salvioli *(22)*; and Spano *(23)*.

Some countries have chosen various policy options to protect older people. For example, in England, the Independent Safeguarding Authority seeks to protect vulnerable adults and ensures by law that employers report a dismissed employee (or volunteer) for causing serious harm to a vulnerable adult, and the employee is then barred from further such employment *(24)*. In Ireland, most local health offices have a dedicated elder maltreatment service with senior caseworkers dealing with elder maltreatment in most local health office areas who work to ensure the safety and well-being of older people while providing support to stop the unwanted behaviour and facilitate the continuation of care. Some countries in the European Region have mandatory reporting of elder maltreatment. This is also the case in the United States, where most states designate certain types of professionals as mandatory reporters of domestic elder maltreatment *(6,25)*.

### *5.2.3 Need for better outcome research and an evaluative framework*

A more scientifically based approach is urgently needed to improve understanding of the scale of the problem, the causes and consequences. Further, more outcome-based research studies are needed to advise policy-makers. This should start with commonly accepted definitions between agencies and longitudinal cohort studies to better understand the risk and protective factors. Research with proper designs is needed to understand the best tools for screening for elder maltreatment in various settings. These may involve a combination of questionnaire designs, record linkage between agencies and clinical algorithms. Research is needed on case identification and adult protection services. Systematic outcome-based evaluation studies are lacking. Various approaches need to be investigated further, such as psychological interventions for perpetrators, educational courses for professionals, public awareness campaigns, school-based intergenerational programmes, programmes that encourage positive attitudes among workers and informal programmes to support caregivers. Information is also needed not only on the costs of elder maltreatment but also on the costs of programmes for preventing it. This report has shown that many programmes are being implemented within the European Region (Box 5.4) but that these should be implemented using an evaluative framework to improve the evidence base.

**Box 5.4. Programming response to elder maltreatment in the WHO European Region**

A survey of health ministry focal people for violence prevention with 40 respondent countries showed that the most frequently implemented interventions at the national level are programmes encouraging positive attitudes towards older people through the use of education programmes for health care workers (24% of countries), supporting victims of maltreatment (24%), respite programmes (22%) and case detection and referral (18%). Of interest, support for informal caregivers (16%) and psychological support programmes for caregivers (8%) were the least frequently implemented. This shows that more widespread implementation needs to occur in the European Region. This presents an opportunity to undertake outcome-based evaluation (Fig. 5.2). Annex 3 presents the full questionnaire.

### *5.2.4 Linking national policy to the momentum of global and European Region policy initiatives*

The Madrid International Plan of Action on Ageing adopted by the Second World Assembly on Ageing in Madrid in 2002 *(27)* recognized the importance of the phenomenon of

**Fig. 5.2. Have the following evidence-based interventions been implemented in your country?**

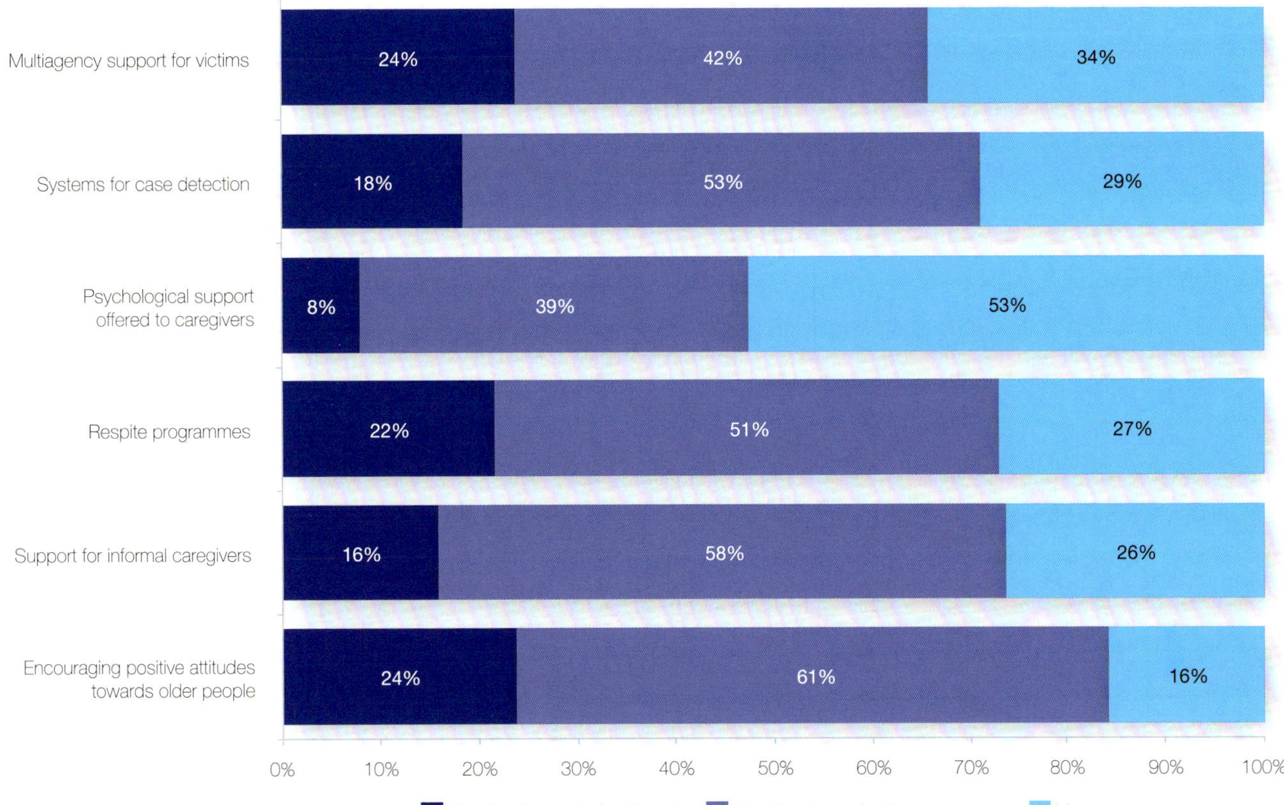


healthy ageing and put it in the framework of the Universal Declaration on Human Rights. The European Commission supported the political message of the Madrid Plan in its communication in March 2002 *(28)*. Further, the Charter of Fundamental Rights of the European Union declares that human dignity is to be protected (Article 1); inhuman or degrading treatment or punishment is to be prohibited (Article 4); and the rights of older people to lead a life of dignity and independence and to participate in social and cultural life (Article 25). The Toronto Declaration on the Global Prevention of Elder Abuse calls on countries to take action for prevention.

The International Network for Prevention of Elder Abuse and Neglect has worked to raise awareness on elder maltreatment with the World Elder Abuse Awareness Day at the global level. This helped to raise awareness and to put the issue on national agendas. The Commission on the Social Determinants of Health has emphasized equity in health and identified older people as a vulnerable group *(29)*. *The Tallinn Charter: Health Systems, Health and Wealth* emphasizes greater equity in health as a fundamental right of all people*(30)*. A resolution of the WHO Regional Committee for Europe *(31)* and the Council of the European Union recommendation on the prevention of injuries *(32)* emphasize a public health approach to preventing violence and injuries and protecting vulnerable groups. These global and European Region policies have helped to promote the priority of the response to elder maltreatment. In a survey of health ministry focal people for violence prevention with 47 respondent countries, only 40% report having a national policy for elder maltreatment *(33)*. This is supported by the findings of a recent global survey of 50 countries emphasizing the need for greater priority to policy *(34)*. Box 5.5 shows examples of various policy approaches. Greater action is needed in the European Region to respond to the problem of elder maltreatment.

## 5.3 Key actions for the WHO European Region

This report recommends nine key action points for Member States for preventing elder maltreatment.

### 1. Develop and implement national policies and plans for preventing elder maltreatment

Health ministries need to take a leadership role in ensuring that national policies and plans for preventing elder maltreatment are developed. These should involve other ministries such as those responsible for justice, education, social welfare, labour, environment and local planning. Efforts should be multidisciplinary with broad representation from other sectors of government and involve nongovernmental organizations and older people *(35)*. Strategies should respond to the needs of older people and promote preventive approaches to maltreatment and also put in place mechanisms for adult protection services. Further, policies

### Box 5.5. Examples of country policies: legislation, regulations, lobbying and advocacy, capacity-building and intersectoral coordination

**Legislation**

- Mandatory reporting laws – Israel, the former Yugoslav Republic of Macedonia
- Law of Violence Prevention in the Family – Israel
- Charters – Germany: Charter of Rights for People in Need of Long-Term Care and Assistance (http://www.pflege-charta.de/en); also a charter in Norway
- Investments in equity – from elder to adult: Adult Protection and Support Act in Scotland
- Only intervening without consent when loss of capacity is proven – England Mental Capacity Act; Israel Law of Guardianship
- Criminal offences – England (MCA) and Scotland (APSA)

**Regulations and guidelines**

- In Spain, Germany, Austria, the Netherlands and Luxembourg – MILCEA (Monitoring in Long-Term Care Pilot Project on Elder Abuse) Project
- Introducing new regulations and protocols for the welfare and health services – Israel: the need to report and intervene
- Introducing new regulations and protocols for institutional services – Israel
- Rolling back – for example, in England, the Independent Safeguarding Authority being cut

**Lobbying and advocacy**

- The lead by nongovernmental organizations – Israel, the former Yugoslav Republic of Macedonia
- In Spain, the Plan Mayores (Plan for Older People)
- Investment in a centre of expertise – Ireland
- Questions about vulnerability – Scotland three-stage test

**Capacity-building**

- Discussion of cash for care (personal budgets, etc., self-directed support) – Austria, Belgium, England and Scotland; the role and extent of monitoring?
- Shifting the focus to empowerment – England: review of No Secrets and a vision for adult social care

**Intersectoral coordination**

- The former Yugoslav Republic of Macedonia – a coordinating body including the welfare services, health services, police and the legal system
- Norway – collaboration between the government and nongovernmental organizations
- Israel – a coordinating forum between welfare services, health services, police and the legal system
- Spain – collaboration between the Ministry of Home Affairs, the Ministry of Justice, trade unions, the Ministry for Equality and the Women's Foundation

should also include providing better support in the community to reduce stress among caregivers. Assessing elder maltreatment nationally is important to determine the prevalence, nature, causes and effects of the various forms of elder maltreatment. Existing policies, laws and regulations should be reviewed and stakeholders and available resources identified *(36)*. Governance mechanisms need to be created to ensure intersectoral action.

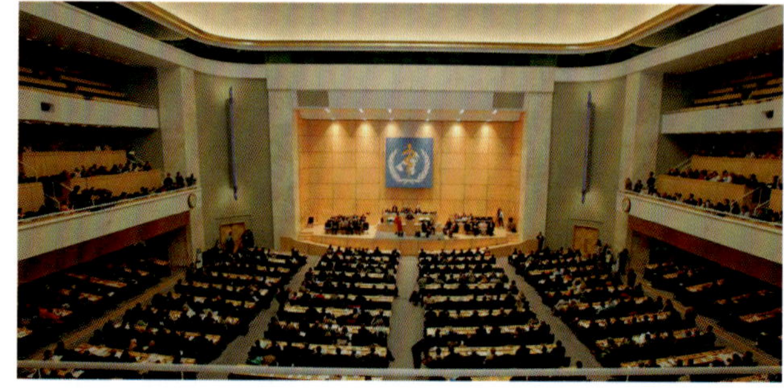

### 2. Take action to improve data on and surveillance of elder maltreatment

This report has shown that routine information on elder maltreatment is inadequate. All levels of data collection need to be improved, and agencies and countries need to share a common definition to better build national and local pictures of the scale of the problem. Reports from the European Region suggest that some data are collected in less than two thirds of the countries. Further, policy-makers and research commissioners may wish to enable researchers and data collectors to share their data more easily. This could apply to findings about the incidence and prevalence of elder maltreatment, and such information would be essential for developing evaluative frameworks for programme implementation (Box 5.6). Information on the costs of maltreatment is also needed. Such data are essential for advocacy. Cross-cultural and cross-national studies are needed to understand the causes of elder maltreatment and to test interventions and theories.

**Box 5.6. An example of policy and service developments following a national prevalence study – the case of Israel**

Findings were presented and discussed at the home of the Israeli President, with top officials from major ministries and nongovernmental organizations present. It received very wide press coverage *(9)*. A national forum for interorganizational coordination was then established, initiated by the Ministry of Social Affairs. JDC-ESHEL, the largest nongovernmental organization, served as a catalyst for governmental policy-makers and organizations serving older people. The emphasis is on multisectoral and multidisciplinary collaboration.

Programmes were developed for community service models of intervention and prevention, special units on the response to elder maltreatment were established within local municipalities. New regulations and protocols were introduced for the welfare departments in each municipality and for long-term care facilities for frail older people.

Work was begun towards developing closer collaboration with the police and the legal system. New regulations and protocols were introduced for general hospitals, long-term care institutions and community health organizations – establishing "violence committees" in each health organization.

A helpline was established for victims of elder maltreatment. Training programmes and case materials were developed for professionals and volunteers. Knowledge and information on elder maltreatment has been developed in Israel, with an emphasis on disseminating knowledge. Data are being systematically collected through special units on elder maltreatment in the community and in health settings, which are required to report any type of abuse or neglect.

### 3. Evaluative research needs to be undertaken as a priority

There is little rigorous knowledge of what works and for whom in preventing elder maltreatment and managing to minimize its harm (see Chapter 4). Systemic responses to primary prevention need to be developed. This is a priority, and good outcome research is needed to improve the evidence base in the European Region and globally. Researchers, donors and policy-makers need to intensify their efforts and make resources available to move the field ahead. Much of this effort should be invested in primary prevention. Older people have suffered in part because the various policy and programmatic solutions related to elder maltreatment were developed to address the maltreatment of children, women or simply "helpless people", rather than being specifically designed to meet the needs of older people. Models developed to help children in distress or to aid women who experience family violence have been applied automatically to older people without conducting any form of independent assessment.

### 4. Responses for victims need to be strengthened

High-quality services need to be provided for victims of maltreatment. Health systems need to be strengthened to provide high-quality primary care services for the detection, management and referral of cases *(11)*. This includes emergency medical services and supporting and rehabilitating victims to address both the physical and mental effects of violence. Better detection of maltreatment, referral to appropriate services, providing social support and protection and preventing repeat perpetration and victimization are all essential to improving the quality of services from the health, justice, education and social sectors. Achieving this requires good coordination between the various actors that would constitute effective adult protection services.

### 5. Build capacity and exchange good practices across the sectors

Ensuring a supply of trained and experienced personnel who are well versed with detection and care is an essential part of an adequate health system response. Educating professionals to recognize, treat and advocate for services to tackle elder maltreatment is important *(26)*. Networks such as health ministry focal people, nongovernmental organizations and academe can disseminate good practices. Capacity building and disseminating good practices are also essential for the justice, education and social care sectors. Older people need to be actively engaged in developing curricula. International agencies such as WHO can facilitate the sharing of examples of best practices throughout the European Region.

**6. Address inequity in the maltreatment of older people**

The economic recession in Europe, the longer life expectancy and ageing population, the strain on social support services and increasing economic pressures on families and older people are exacerbating the vulnerability of older people to maltreatment. Equity needs to be incorporated into all levels of government policy to address this cause of social injustice. WHO's Health 2020 approach to a new health policy framework for the European Region and the recommendations of the WHO Commission on Social Determinants of Health *(29)* emphasize that all social and economic policy needs to be equitable and incorporate health as a key outcome. The health sector has a key role to advocate for this across other government departments and to highlight elder maltreatment as an effect of social policies. As part of this, policies and programmes should address gender inequity associated with the different types of violence. Further, some policies, such as those for universal health care, social care and protection, should seek to look after disadvantaged people. The health sector needs to ensure that the prevention of maltreatment is universally incorporated into primary health care services and can support community-based action, focusing special attention on socially disadvantaged areas. Engagement with older people and civil society is essential to a whole-community coordination approach using community development principles.

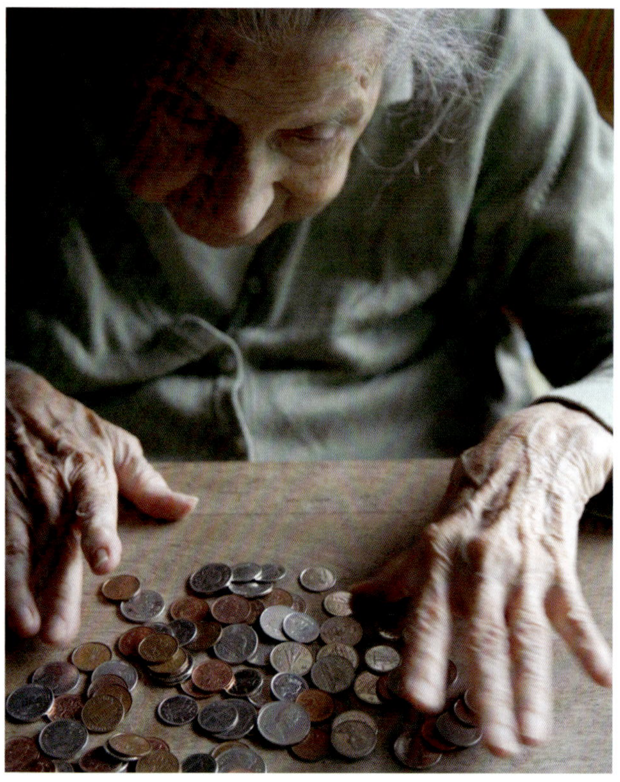

**7. Raise awareness and target investment for preventing elder maltreatment**

Raising awareness that maltreatment among older people should be prevented is paramount. *Missing voices (37)*, developed by WHO and the International Network for the Prevention of Elder Abuse, gathered qualitative information on elder maltreatment and has done much to advocate for this. The initial focus has been on protecting older people's dignity and their right not to be maltreated. Advocates for preventing maltreatment among older people are needed throughout the European Region. Potential targets for advocacy are politicians, policy-makers, funding agencies, health and other professionals, the mass media and older people themselves. International and national nongovernmental organizations, the health sector and other sectors need to advocate for broad government policy leading to safer environments in social, community and family settings. Social marketing, mass media and education programmes should be used to raise awareness of the effects of maltreatment and to promote a healthy-ageing approach to overcome negative stereotyping. Engaging older people in these processes, including in making laws, is essential to this process.

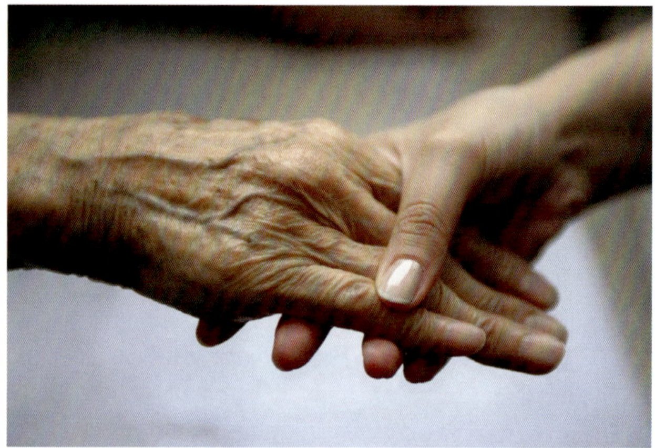

**8. Protective factors, a life-course approach and intergenerational cohesion**

The demographic revolution in the European Region is accompanied by profound changes and presents fundamental challenges to social integration, to social protection and social policies. Such a situation creates sociopolitical and policy challenges to social cohesion and to the social fabric of societies. A generational contract and innovative policy responses are therefore needed at the individual, familial and societal levels, with special emphasis on prevention. Innovative approaches to reducing social isolation through the use of technologies such as the Internet would allow older people to say in touch and avoid isolation. Relating to the different stages along the life course and how they affect family and care relations should be advocated. Reducing ageism and increasing the perceived value of older people in society would be part of this. Ethnic and cultural norms should be considered when developing programmes in this field, and cultural diversity should be more deeply researched *(10,38)*.

**9. Ethics and the quality of services in the community and in institutions**

The health and social sectors provide care for older people and oversee ethical standards and the quality of care for older people. The Charter of Rights for People in Need of Long-Term Care and Assistance adopted in Germany in 2007 demonstrated one such approach. Such charters provide standards that are binding for the organization of high-quality care. Continuous quality improvement for the entire care and support sector is emphasized. Quality assurance and other organizational mechanisms need to be put in place to protect older people by ensuring that quality standards are met.

## 5.4 Conclusions

Elder maltreatment is pervasive in all countries in the European Region. Conservative estimates suggest that at least 4 million people experience it in any one year. The full scale of the problem is not properly understood, but it has far-reaching consequences for the mental and physical well-being of tens of millions of older people and results in their premature death. Maltreatment has been shown to be a public health and societal priority in the Region. Despite this, few countries have devoted adequate resources to studying its scale, causes and consequences and what can be done to prevent it. Given this inadequate response, this report proposes a set of actions for Member States, international agencies, nongovernmental organizations and other stakeholders. This report has outlined the great burden of maltreatment among older people and some of its causes and has highlighted promising prevention programmes. A strong argument is made for advocating for increased investment in research, prevention and protection. Prevention can only be achieved by being mainstreamed into other areas of health and social policy. Awareness of the problem is increasing, and the public is increasingly demanding action. This report has proposed an approach that is strong in prevention and evaluation. There is an urgent need to protect older people and work towards prevention.

The prevention of elder maltreatment has reached a crossroads. It has been identified as a serious threat, and more resources are needed to understand its causes and how to prevent it. Elder maltreatment is unacceptable – older people are entitled to the best quality of life, free from abuse and neglect. This report calls on policy-makers and practitioners to commit to achieve this end.

## 5.5 References


1. Lowenstein A, Katz R, Gur-Yaish N. Cross-national variations in elder care: antecedents and outcomes. In: Szinovacz ME, Davey A, eds. *Caregiving contexts: cultural, familial and societal implications*. New York, Springer, 2008:93–114.
2. Schneider JW. Social problems theory: the constructionist view. *Annual Review of Sociology*, 1985, 11:209–229.
3. Spector M, Kitsuse JI. *Constructing social problems*. New York, Transaction Publishers, 2000.
4. European Commission. Health and long-term care in the European Union. *Eurobarometer*, 2007, 283.
5. Preventing elder abuse: can we learn from child protection? *Lancet*, 2011, 377:876.
6. *Demography report 2008: meeting social needs in an ageing society.* Brussels, European Commission, 2008.
7. Bengtson VL. Beyond the nuclear family: the increasing importance of multigenerational bonds. *Journal of Marriage and the Family*, 2000, 63:1–16.
8. Stuckler D et al. The public health effect of economic crises and alternative policy responses in Europe: an empirical analysis. *Lancet*, 2009, 374:315–323.
9. Lowenstein A. Global ageing and the challenges to families. In: Johnson M et al., eds. *Cambridge handbook of age and ageing*. Cambridge, Cambridge University Press, 2005:403–413.
10. Aneshensel CS. *Profiles in caregiving: the unexpected carer*. Cambridge, Cambridge University Press, 1995.
11. Krug E et al., eds. *World report on violence and health*. Geneva, World Health Organization, 2002 (http://www.who.int/violence_injury_prevention/violence/world_report/en, accessed 9 May 2011).
12. Bonnie R, Wallace R, eds. *Elder mistreatment: abuse, neglect, and exploitation in an aging America.* Washington, DC, National Academies Press, 2003.
13. Brammer A, Biggs S. *Define elder abuse.* Journal of Social Welfare and Family Law, 1998, 20:285–304.
14. Quinn MJ, Heisler CJ. The legal response to elder abuse and neglect. *Journal of Elder Abuse and Neglect*, 2002, 14:61–77.
15. *Interpersonal violence against women throughout the life span*. Washington, DC, American College of Obstetricians and Gynecologists, 2009 (http://www.acog.org/departments/dept_notice.cfm?recno=17&bulletin=186, accessed 9 May 2011).

16. *Understanding elder maltreatment. Fact sheet 2010*. Atlanta, United States Centers for Disease Control and Prevention, 2010 (http://www.cdc.gov/violenceprevention/pdf/em-factsheet-a.pdf, accessed 9 May 2011).

17. Manthorpe J et al. *Secondary data analysis of data on elder abuse: a report for the Department of Health*. London, Social Care Workforce Research Unit, 2011.

18. *Macedonia in figures 2010*. Skopje, State Statistical Office, the former Yugoslav Republic of Macedonia, 2010.

19. *Report on violence and health in Macedonia and guide for prevention*. Skopje, Ministry of Health, the former Yugoslav Republic of Macedonia, 2006.

20. *Annual report 2010*. Skopje, Ministry of Labor and Social Policy, the former Yugoslav Republic of Macedonia.

21. Mestheneos E, Triantafillou J. *Supporting family carers of older people in Europe. The pan-European background report*. Athens, EUROFAMCARE, 2005 (http://www.sextant.gr/docs/EFCpeubare_051006_a5.pdf, accessed 9 May 2011).

22. Savioli G. *Gli anziani e le badanti* [Old people and the minders]. Giornale di Gerontologia, 2007, 55:59–61.

23. Spano P. *L e convenienze nascoste. Il fenomeno delle badanti e le risposte del welfare.* [The hidden conveniences. The phenomenon of caregivers and the responses of welfare.] Portogruaro, Nuova Dimensione, Ediciclo, 2006.

24. Hussein S et al. Banned from working in social care: secondary analysis of staff characteristics and reasons for their referrals to the POVA List in England and Wales. *Health and Social Care in the Community*, 2009, 17:423–433.

25. *The National Elder Abuse Incidence Study*. Newark, DE, National Center on Elder Abuse at the American Public Human Services Association in Collaboration with Westat, Inc., 1998 (http://aoa.gov/AoA_Programs/Elder_Rights/Elder_Abuse/docs/ABuseReport_Full.pdf, accessed 9 May 2011).

26. Payne BK. Training adult protective service workers about domestic violence: training needs and strategies. *Journal of Violence against Women*, 2008, 14:1199–1213.

27. *Report of the Second World Assembly on Ageing, Madrid, 8–12 April 2002*. New York, United Nations, 2002 (http://daccess-dds-ny.un.org/doc/UNDOC/GEN/N02/397/51/PDF/N0239751.pdf?OpenElement, accessed 9 May 2011).

28. *Europe's response to world ageing: promoting economic and social progress in an ageing world. A contribution of the European Commission to the Second World Assembly on Ageing*. Brussels, European Commission, 2002 (COM(2002) 143).

29. Commission on Social Determinants of Health. *Closing the gap in a generation: health equity through action on the social determinants of health. Final report of the Commission on Social Determinants of Health*. Geneva, World Health Organization, 2008 (http://www.who.int/social_determinants/resources/gkn_lee_al.pdf, accessed 9 May 2011).

30. *The Tallinn Charter: Health Systems for Health and Wealth*. Copenhagen, WHO Regional Office for Europe, 2008 (http://www.euro.who.int/__data/assets/pdf_file/0008/886613/E91438.pdf, accessed 9 May 2011).

31. WHO Regional Committee for Europe. *Resolution EUR/RC55/R9 on prevention of injuries in the WHO European Region*. Copenhagen, WHO Regional Office for Europe, 2005 (http://www.euro.who.int/__data/assets/pdf_file/0017/88100/RC55_eres09.pdf, accessed 9 May 2011).

32. European Council. Council recommendation of 31 May 2007 on the prevention of injury and promotion of safety. *Official Journal of the European Union*, 2007, 200 C:1–2.

33. Sethi D et al. *Preventing injuries in Europe: from international collaboration to local implementation*. Copenhagen, WHO Regional Office for Europe, 2010 (http://www.euro.who.int/en/what-we-publish/abstracts/preventing-injuries-in-europe-from-international-collaboration-to-local-implementation, accessed 9 May 2011).

34. Podnieks E et al. WorldView Environmental Scan on Elder Abuse. *Journal of Elder Abuse and Neglect*, 2010, 22:164–179.

35. Naughton C et al. *Abuse and neglect of older people in Ireland: report on the National Study of Elder Abuse and Neglect*. Dublin, University College Dublin, 2010.

36. *Preventing injuries and violence: a guide for ministries of health*. Geneva, World Health Organization, 2007 (http://www.who.int/violence_injury_prevention/publications/injury_policy_planning/prevention_moh/en/index.html, accessed 9 May 2011).

37. WHO and INPEA. *Missing voices: views of older persons on elder abuse*. Geneva, World Health Organization, 2002 (http://www.who.int/ageing/projects/elder_abuse/missing_voices/en, accessed 9 May 2011).

38. Kosberg J. Study of elder abuse within diverse cultures. *Journal of Elder Abuse and Neglect*, 2005, 15:71–90.

# Annex 1. Methods used

## Background on statistical information

This report relies on several WHO sources of information for the statistical data, tables, figures and annexes: a) the WHO Global Burden of Disease 2004 *(1)*, b) the WHO European Health for All mortality database *(2)*, c) the WHO detailed mortality *(3)* and hospital admission *(4)* databases. WHO data for the European Region are collected every six months.

## How can violence be measured?

Deaths and health states from violence are categorically attributed to one underlying cause using the rules and conventions of the International Classification of Diseases (ICD) *(5,6)*. ICD-10 codes, which are not available for all the countries, were used for specific causes, as reported in Table 1, for age groups 60 years and older. ICD-9 and ICD-10 codes were used for data on all homicides for age groups 65 years and older. Table 1 shows the ICD codes used for assaults.

## Global Burden of Disease database

The Global Burden of Disease database *(1)* combines mortality data derived from national vital registration systems with information obtained from surveys, censuses, epidemiological studies and health service data. It represents the most comprehensive view of global mortality and morbidity available today. The Global Burden of Disease data are disaggregated into six geographical WHO regions and 14 subregions. The estimates provided are for the year 2004. The cause list used for the Global Burden of Disease 2004 project has four levels of disaggregation that include 135 specific diseases and injuries.

Overall mortality is divided into three broad groups of causes:

A. Group I: communicable diseases, maternal causes, conditions arising in the perinatal period and nutritional deficiencies;

B. Group II: noncommunicable diseases; and

C. Group III: intentional and unintentional injuries, with external cause codes;

Disability-adjusted life-years (DALYS) have been used to quantify the loss of healthy life due to injury or disease. This measure is a composite score of both the years of life lost due to premature death and the years of life lived with disability. One DALY lost is one year of healthy life lost, either due to premature death or disability.

The Global Burden of Disease data were used to calculate rates and rate ratios.

## WHO European Health for All database (off-line version, July 2010)

The WHO European Health for All database *(7)* contains data on health and population indicators for the 53 countries belonging to the WHO European Region. Data on life expectancy at birth and at 65 years of age, by sex and country, were retrieved from this source and were used in charts showing:

- the gap of life expectancy at birth between the two sexes; and
- the changes in life expectancy at 65 years of age between 1990 and 2008 (or last available year) by sex and country.

Countries below the diagonal lines are those for which life expectancy at 65 years decreased in that period of time (Annex 2, Fig. 5).

## WHO European Health for All database (HFA-MDB): mortality supplement by 67 causes of death, age and sex (off-line version, July 2010)

The WHO European Health for All database contains data on health indicators, including mortality, morbidity and disability from multiple causes, including external causes of injuries *(2)*. These data allow trend analysis and international comparisons for several health statistics. These data also contain age-standardized mortality indicators. Age-standardized rates per 100 000 population in the European Region are presented by sex and for the age groups 0–4, 5–14, 15–29, 30–44, 45–59 and 60–74 years, 65 years or older and 75 years or older. Data are compiled, validated and processed uniformly to improve the international comparability of statistics. Data available are from 1979 onwards. This report used the version of the Health for All database dated July 2010.

Data on population were retrieved from the Health for All database *(7)* and were used to calculate demographic statistics:

- the ageing index: the number of people aged 65 years and older per 100 population; and

**Table 1. External causes of injury and their corresponding ICD codes**

| Type of violence | ICD-9 code | ICD-10 code |
|---|---|---|
| Interpersonal violence | E950–E968 | X85–Y09 |
| Poisoning and other substances | | X85–X90 |
| Assault by drugs, medicaments and biological substances | | X85 |
| Assault by corrosive substance | | X86 |
| Assault by pesticides | | X87 |
| Assault by gases and vapours | | X88 |
| Assault by other specified chemicals and noxious substances | | X89 |
| Assault by unspecified chemical or noxious substance | | X90 |
| Hanging, strangulation and drowning | | X91–X92 |
| Assault by hanging, strangulation and suffocation | E963 | X91 |
| Assault by drowning and submersion | E964 | X92 |
| Handgun, firearm and explosive material | E965 | X93–X96 |
| Assault by handgun discharge | | X93 |
| Assault by rifle, shotgun and larger firearm discharge | | X94 |
| Assault by other and unspecified firearm discharge | | X95 |
| Assault by explosive material | | X96 |
| Assault with sharp objects | E966 | X99 |
| Assault with blunt objects | | Y00 |
| Assault (sexual or not) by bodily force | E960 | Y04–Y05 |
| Assault by bodily force | | Y04 |
| Sexual assault by bodily force | | Y05 |
| Neglect, abandonment and other maltreatment syndromes | | Y06–Y07 |
| Neglect and abandonment | | Y06 |
| Other maltreatment syndromes | | Y07 |
| Other means, specified | | X97–X98, Y01–Y03, Y08 |
| Assault by smoke, fire and flames | | X97 |
| Assault by steam, hot vapours and hot objects | | X98 |
| Assault by pushing from high place | | Y01 |
| Assault by pushing or placing victim before moving object | | Y02 |
| Assault by crashing of motor vehicle | | Y03 |
| Assault by other specified means | | Y08 |
| Assault by unspecified means | E968 | Y09 |

- the old-age dependency index: the population aged 65 years and older per 100 population of working age (15–64 years).

The old-age dependency index measures the extent to which the working population of a country has to support older people. The higher the index, the higher the dependence (Annex 2, Fig. 2).

**Table 2. ICD codes for analysis of assaults by cause**

| Causes | ICD-10 codes |
|---|---|
| Poisoning | X85–X90 |
| Hanging and drowning | X91–X92 |
| Firearm | X93–X96 |
| Sharp object | X99 |
| Blunt object | Y00 |
| Bodily force including sexual | Y04–Y05 |
| Neglect | Y06–Y07 |
| Other assaults, specified means | X97–X98, Y01–Y03, Y08 |
| Other assaults, unspecified means | Y09 |

## WHO European detailed mortality (and hospital admissions) database

The WHO European detailed mortality database *(3)* is the more complete mortality data source for the European Region. It includes, for the available countries, mortality data by five-year age groups in ICD-9, ICD-10 and MTL code officially reported by WHO Member States. The data are available from 1990 onwards. For the purposes of this report, data were downloaded for 2006–2008 (or the most recent three years) for people aged 60 years and older. Data with similar age bands are also available for hospital admissions but only for a limited number of countries *(4)*. This report used the July 2010 update of the detailed mortality (and hospital admissions) database. Data were also analysed by mode of homicide and are presented in Fig. 2.4 and Annex 2, Fig. 4.

## The EU Injury Database

The EU Injury Database *(8)* provides data on emergency department attendance for selected hospitals from several countries.

## Additional population data

To forecast population trends from 2010 to 2050, data from the Population Division of the United Nations Department of Economic and Social Affairs *(9)* were retrieved, summed for each Member State and then grouped.

## Confidence intervals

Except for the confidence interval of the study from United Kingdom, given the large sample size, the 95% confidence intervals shown in Fig. 2.7 have been calculated with standard methods, assuming normal distribution *(10)*.

## Limitations of current routine information systems

These data have several limitations.

First, vital registration data are missing in a few European Region countries. This is particularly the case in some of the countries affected by transition and conflict. Mortality data are also not adequate for Andorra, Monaco and Turkey.

Second, the Global Burden of Disease 2004 estimates are based on extrapolations of information compiled to estimate the burden of disease. Although these have been updated using more recent studies than those in 1990, those measuring disability are still few.

Third, DALYs do not capture data on all the health effects of injury. For example, they do not account for the mental and reproductive health effects of violence or injuries.

Fourth, since systems and practices for recording and handling health data vary between countries, the availability and accuracy of the data reported to WHO may be variable.

Fifth, the data are prone to sociocultural contexts, and intentional injuries may be misclassified as unintentional or of undetermined intent. International comparisons between countries and their interpretation should thus be carried out with caution.

Sixth, few countries provided reliable morbidity data to WHO information systems – the regional picture is incomplete.

## The WHO survey questionnaire on prevention of elder maltreatment

WHO prepared a brief questionnaire on elder maltreatment with the advice of an expert panel. This was piloted and then modified. The questionnaire has items on the scale of the problem, the policy response and implementation of evidence-informed programmes for preventing elder maltreatment. The latter were selected after reviewing the literature and with the input of the expert panel *(11,12)*. The questionnaire (Annex 3) was sent to 46 health ministry focal people on violence prevention, who answered the questions in collaboration with

10. Clopper C, Pearson ES. The use of confidence or fiducial limits illustrated in the case of the binomial. *Biometrika* 1934, 26:404–413.

11. *Preventing injuries and violence: a guide for ministries of health*. Geneva, World Health Organization, 2007 (http://www.who.int/violence_injury_prevention/publications/injury_policy_planning/prevention_moh/en/index.html, accessed 9 May 2011).

12. Wood S et al. *Elder abuse. A review of evidence for prevention*. Liverpool, Liverpool John Moores University, 2010 (http://www.cph.org.uk/showPublication.aspx?pubid=672, accessed 9 May 2011).

13. *Healthy life expectancy (HALE) at birth (years)*. Geneva, WHO Statistical Information System (WHOSIS), 2007 (http://www.who.int/whosis/indicators/2007HALE0/en, accessed 9 May 2011).

# Annex 2. Additional results

**Fig. 1. Healthy life expectancy (HALE) at birth in years, WHO European Region, 2007**

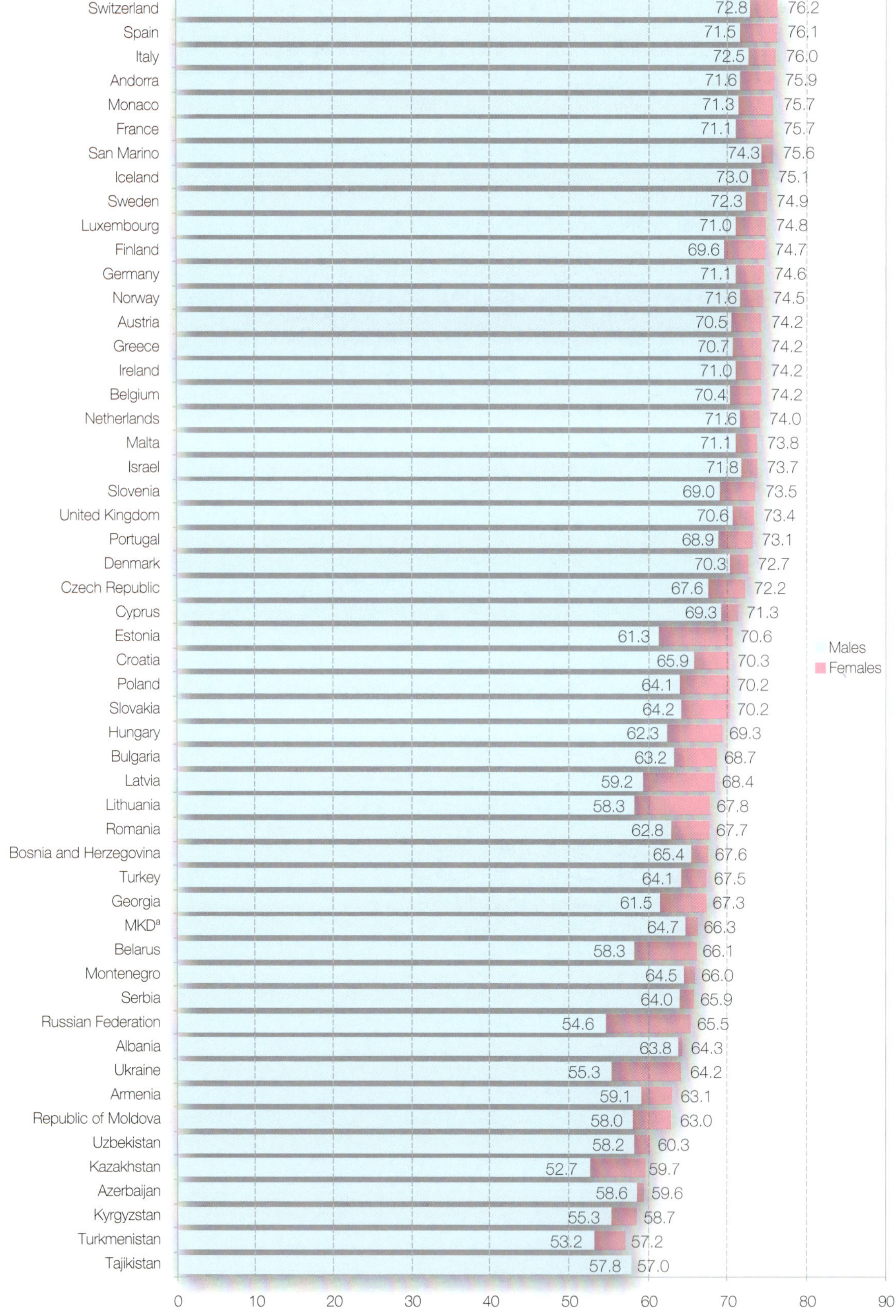


[a] MKD stands for the former Yugoslav Republic of Macedonia; it is an abbreviation of the International Organization for Standardization (ISO), not WHO.

*Source: World health statistics 2009 (1).*

**Fig. 2. Old-age dependency ratio for countries in the WHO European Region: the number of people aged 65 years and older per 100 people 15–64 years old**

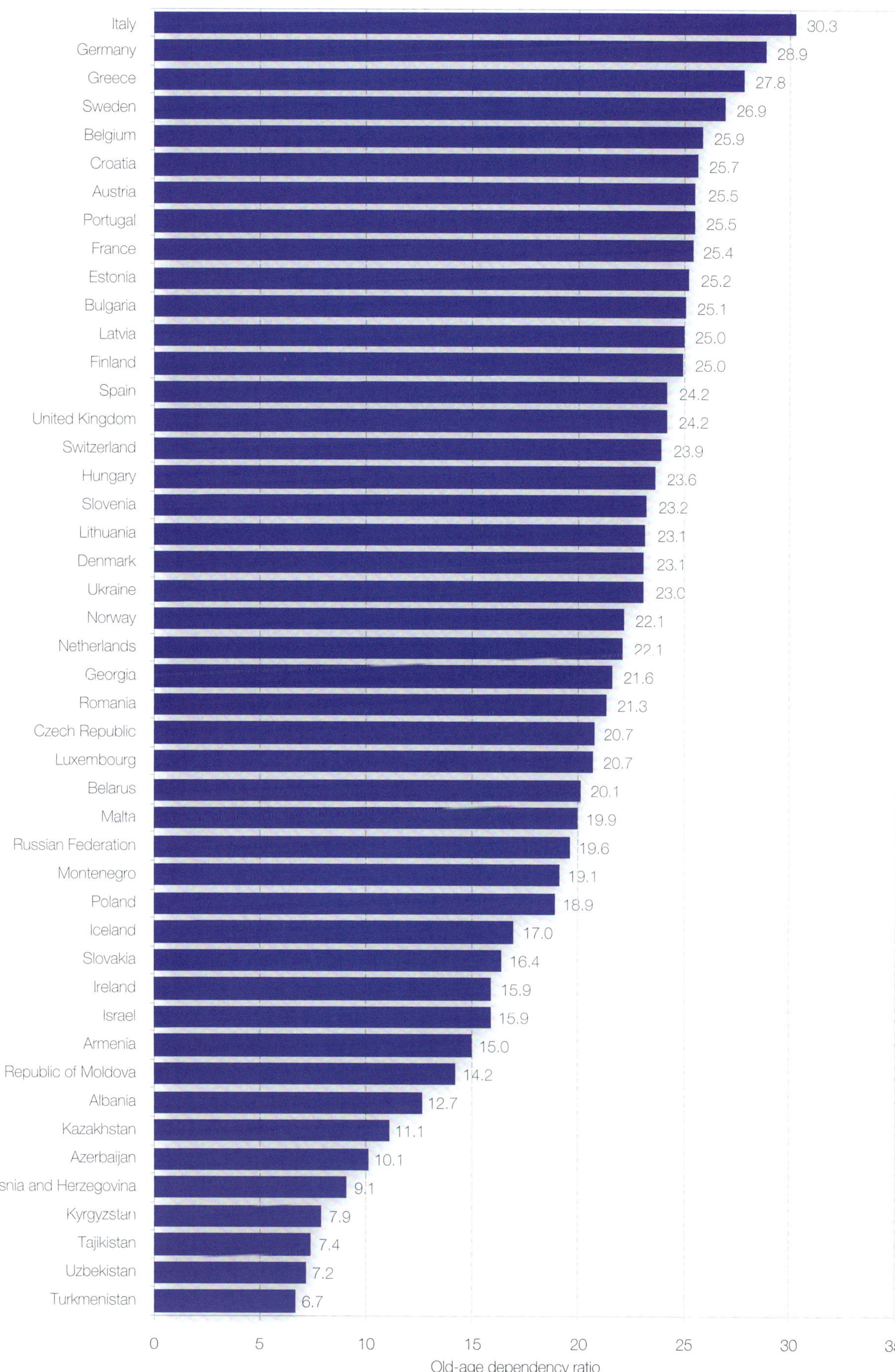


*Source:* European Health for All database *(2)*.

**Fig. 3. Distribution of DALYs lost from various causes of unintentional and intentional injuries among people aged 60 years and older**

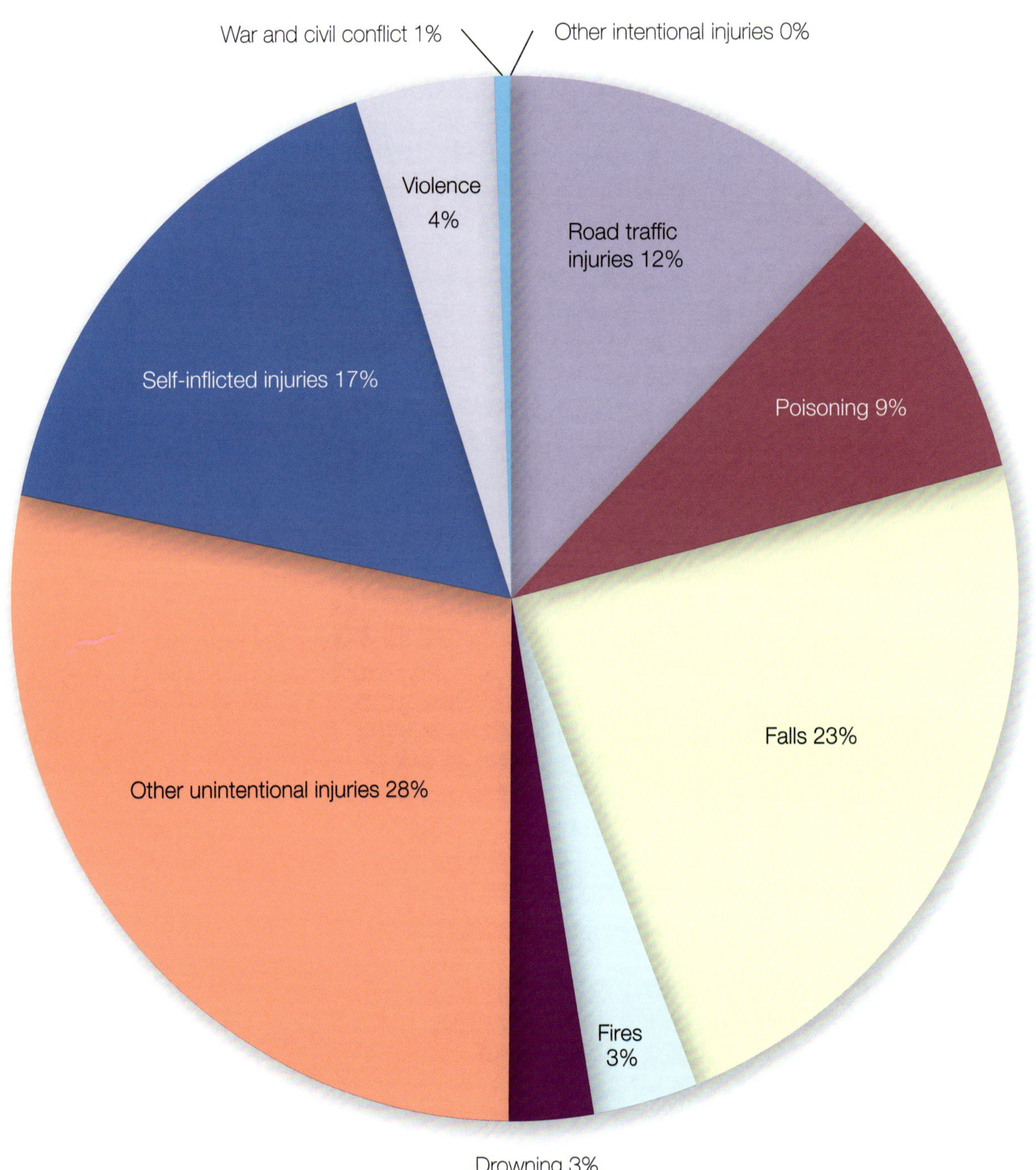


*Source: The global burden of disease: 2004 update (3).*

**Fig. 4. Proportion of all homicides among victims aged 60 years and older perpetrated using sharp weapons, strangulation, firearms and other means in selected countries in the WHO European Region, average for 2005–2007 or last available three years**

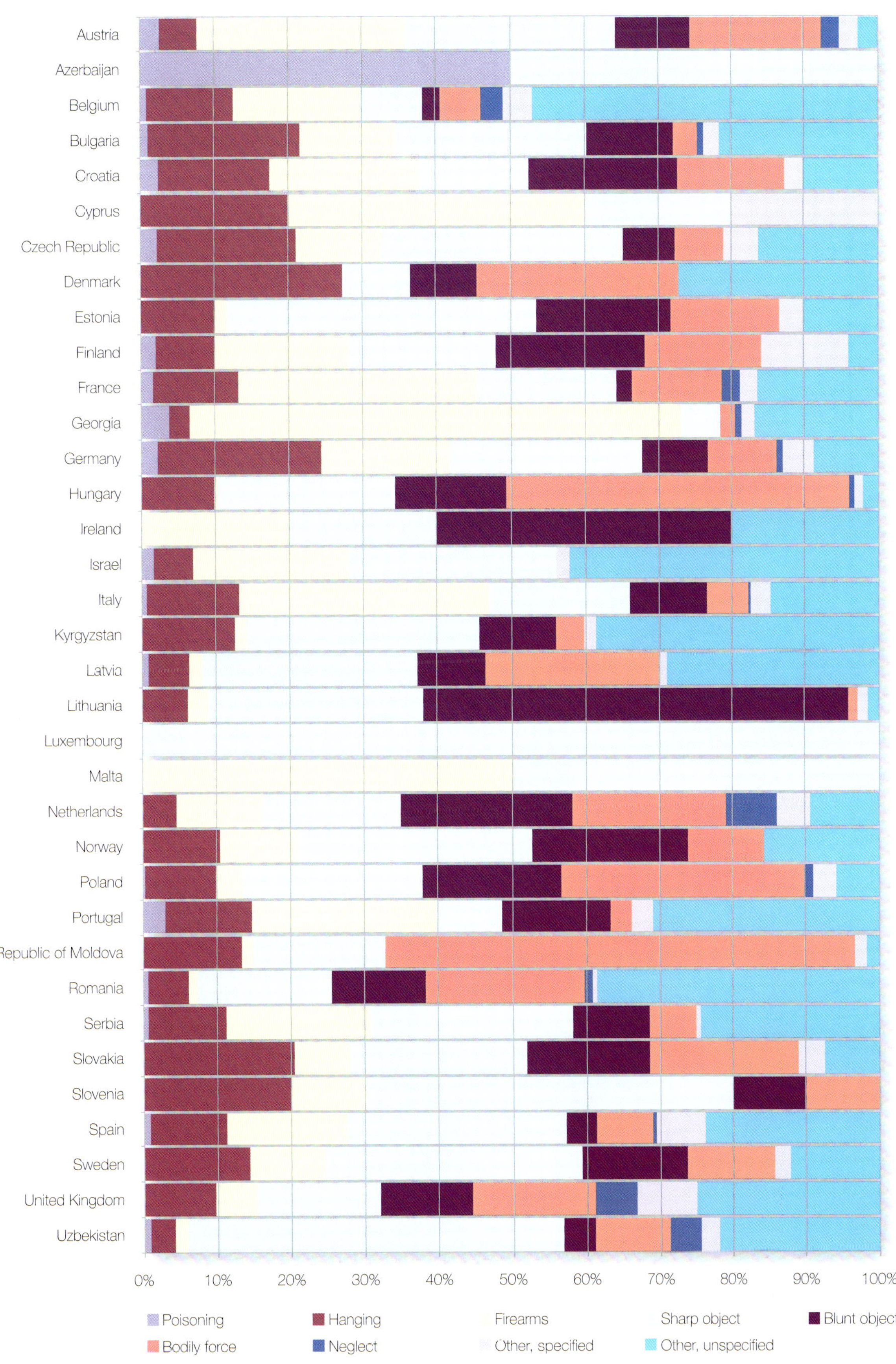


*Source*: European detailed mortality database *(4)*.

**Fig. 5. Proportion of the population of both sexes aged 65 years and older in countries and country groups, 1990 and 2008 (or last available year)**

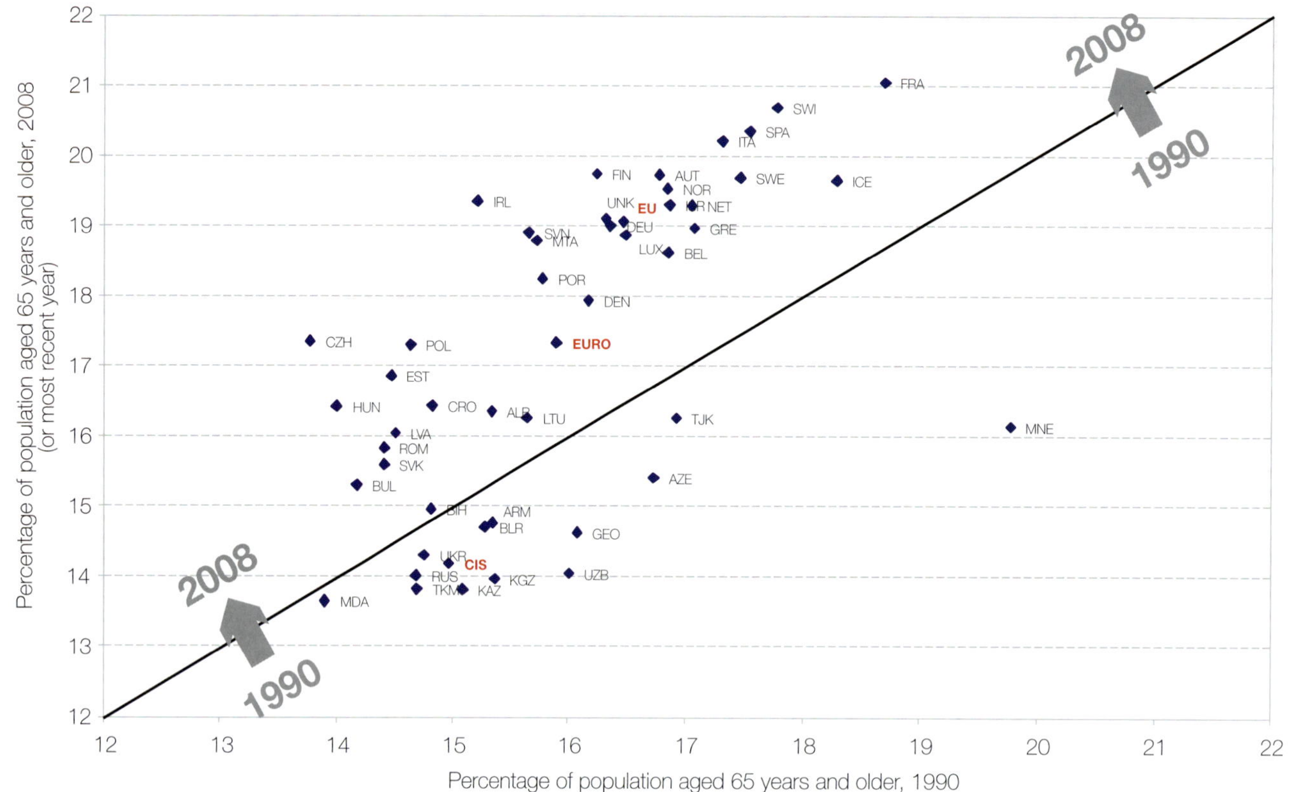


*Source*: European Health for All database *(2)*.

ALB: Albania; AND: Andorra; ARM: Armenia; AUT: Austria; AZE: Azerbaijan; BEL: Belgium; BLR: Belarus; BIH: Bosnia and Herzegovina; BUL: Bulgaria; CIS: average for CIS countries; CRO: Croatia; CYP: Cyprus; CZH: Czech Republic; DEN: Denmark; DEU: Germany; EST: Estonia; EU: average for EU countries; EURO: average for European Region; FIN: Finland; FRA: France; GEO: Georgia; GRE: Greece; HUN: Hungary; ICE: Iceland; IRE: Ireland; ISR: Israel; ITA: Italy; KAZ: Kazakhstan; KGZ: Kyrgyzstan; LTU: Lithuania; LVA: Latvia; LUX: Luxembourg; MAT: Malta; MDA: Republic of Moldova; MKD[a]: The former Yugoslav Republic of Macedonia; MNE: Montenegro; MON: Monaco; NET: Netherlands; NOR: Norway; POL: Poland; POR: Portugal; ROM: Romania; RUS: Russian Federation; SMR: San Marino; SPA: Spain; SRB: Serbia; SVK: Slovakia; SVN: Slovenia; SWE: Sweden; SWI: Switzerland; TJK: Tajikistan; TKM: Turkmenistan; TUR: Turkey; UKR: Ukraine; UNK: United Kingdom; UZB: Uzbekistan.

Countries above the line have shown increases in the proportion of people aged 65 years and older since 1990, whereas those below the line have reported a fall since 1990.

[a] MKD stands for the former Yugoslav Republic of Macedonia; it is an abbreviation of the International Organization for Standardization (ISO), not WHO.

**Table 3. Selected studies of the prevalence of self-reported elder maltreatment reported by family caregivers, WHO European Region**

| Location | Population under study | Maltreatment measure | Prevalence period | Prevalence of maltreatment | Details | Reference |
|---|---|---|---|---|---|---|
| Spain | 789 interviews of adults who dedicate themselves to caring for older people (private homes); proportional sample at the national level | Face-to-face interview | One year | 4.6% | Physical 1.8%, mental 1.8%, neglect 0.4%, financial 1.9%, sexual 0.1% | *(5)* |
| Spain | 789 interviews of adults who dedicate themselves to caring for older people who are dependent (physically or intellectually) to a lesser or greater degree in private homes; proportional sample of dependent people at the national level | Face-to-face interview | One year | 5.7% | Physical 2.4%, mental 2.4%, neglect 0.5%, financial 2.4% | *(5)* |
| United Kingdom, Northern Ireland | Referrals to Northern Ireland Community Mental Health Team: aged 65+ years, DSM-III-R dementia, community-dwelling, and main caregiver; 38 older people | Not standard | One year | 37% | Physical 11%, verbal 34% | *(6)* |
| Israel | 24 800 older people: men older than 65 years and women older than 60 years referred to Israel social services after social worker training in 2002 | Social worker reported abuse or neglect | One year | 0.5% incidence | | *(7)* |
| United Kingdom, Essex and London | 220 family caregivers of people newly referred to secondary psychiatric services with dementia who were living at home | Cross-sectional survey: modified Conflict Tactics Scales | Three months | 52% of caregivers reported some abusive behaviour | 34% of caregivers reported important levels of maltreatment; verbal abuse was most commonly reported; only 1.4% of caregivers reported occasional physical abuse | *(8)* |
| United Kingdom, London | Caregivers (51) of older receiving and consecutively referred for geriatric services respite care, or attending day hospital for respite | Not standard | One year | Any (physical, verbal or neglect): 45% | 27% of caregivers admitted to one type of abuse, 14% to two types and 3% to all three types of abuse | *(9)* |
| United Kingdom | 67 caregivers recruited from a voluntary organization for dementia caregivers | Not standard | One year | Any: 55% | Verbal 52%, physical 12% | *(10)* |
| Netherlands, Amsterdam | People with dementia diagnosed according to CAMDEX and DSM-III-R criteria (n = 169) recruited from an Amsterdam epidemiological study, day hospital and memory clinic; caregivers provided direct care at least once every two weeks | Own questions | One year | | Verbal 30.2%, physical 10.7% | *(11)* |

**Table 3. Selected studies of the prevalence of self-reported elder maltreatment reported by family caregivers, WHO European Region**

| Location | Population under study | Maltreatment measure | Prevalence period | Prevalence of maltreatment | Details | Reference |
|---|---|---|---|---|---|---|
| United Kingdom London | People aged 65+ years with a DSM-III-R dementia diagnosis (82) and the main co-resident caregivers were recruited from a London Health authority registry and dementia community support team | Conflict Tactics Scales and own items | One year | Any: 52% | Verbal 51%, physical 20% | *(12)* |
| Sweden, Stockholm | People aged 74+ years living in an institution or at home and caregivers; 219 family members of cognitively impaired older people (case group) and 255 family members of cognitively healthy older (control group) were interviewed about their situation as a caregiver to an old person | Qualitative interview | Not stated | Any: 12% | | *(13)* |
| Spain, five municipalities (Vitoria, Seville, Las Palmas, Telde and San Bartolomé de Tirajana) in Pais Vasco, Andalucia and Canarias | Home-care workers providing service to 2351 dependent older people | A questionnaire was administered to the home-care workers of the social services of the participating municipalities; it was explained to them what the study considered to be neglect and abuse; prevalence period not stated | Not stated | 4.7% | 81% of victims were women; the main type of maltreatment detected was neglect | *(14)* |

## Emergency department attendances for assaults in older people

The EU Injury Database provides the following estimate: there are about 105 000 assaults per year among people aged 60 years and older in EU countries (hospital treated) *(15)*. The estimate is based on 976 actual EU Injury Database cases in seven countries: Austria, Cyprus, Germany, Latvia, Netherlands, Slovenia and Sweden (Robert Bauer, Austrian Road Safety Board, personal communication, 2011).

## References


1. *World health statistics 2009*. Geneva, World Health Organization, 2009 (http://www.who.int/whosis/whostat/en, accessed 9 May 2011).

2. European Health for All database [online database]. Copenhagen, WHO Regional Office for Europe, 2010 (http://www.euro.who.int/hfadb, accessed 9 May 2011).

3. *The global burden of disease: 2004 update*. Geneva, World Health Organization, 2008 (http://www.who.int/healthinfo/global_burden_disease/2004_report_update/en/index.html, accessed 9 May 2011).

4. European detailed mortality database (DMDB) [online database]. Copenhagen, WHO Regional Office for Europe, 2010 (http://www.euro.who.int/en/what-wedo/ data-and-evidence/databases, accessed 9 May 2011).

5. Iborra I. *Maltrato de personas mayores en la familia en España [Elder maltreatment within families in Spain]*. Valencia, Queen Sofía Center, 2008 (Serie Documentos No. 13).

6. Compton SA, Flanagan P, Gregg W. Elder abuse in people with dementia in Northern Ireland: prevalence and predictors in cases referred to a psychiatry of old

age service. *International Journal of Geriatric Psychiatry*, 1997, 12:632–635.

7. Iecovich E, Lankri M, Drori D. Elder abuse and neglect – a pilot incidence study in Israel. *Journal of Elder Abuse and Neglect*, 2004, 16(3):45–63.

8. Cooper C et al. Abuse of people with dementia by family carers: representative cross sectional survey. *British Medical Journal*, 2009, 338:b155.

9. Homer AC, Gilleard C. Abuse of elderly people by their carers. *British Medical Journal*, 1990, 301:1359–1362.

10. Cooney C, Mortimer A. Elder abuse and dementia: a pilot study. *International Journal of Social Psychiatry*, 1995, 4:276–283.

11. Pot AM et al. Verbal and physical aggression against demented elderly by informal caregivers in the Netherlands. *Social Psychiatry and Psychiatric Epidemiology,* 1996, 31:156–162.

12. Cooney C, Howard R, Lawlor B. Abuse of vulnerable people with dementia by their carers: can we identify those most at risk? *International Journal of Geriatric Psychiatry*, 2006, 21:564–571.

13. Grafstrom M, Nordberg A, Winblad B. Abuse is in the eye of the beholder. *Scandinavian Journal of Social Medicine*, 1993, 21:247–255.

14. Bazo MT. Negligencia y malos tratos a las personas mayores en España [Neglect and maltreatment of older people in Spain]. *Revista Española Geriatría y Gerontología*, 2001, 36:8–14.

15. EU injury database [online database]. Brussels, European Commission, 2010 (https://webgate.ec.europa.eu/idbpa, accessed 9 May 2011).

# Annex 3. Questionnaire on the prevention of elder maltreatment

## Definition of elder maltreatment

**Elder maltreatment is any abuse and neglect of persons aged 60 and older by a caregiver or another person in a relationship involving an expectation of trust.**

**This includes physical, sexual and psychological abuse, deprivation or neglect and financial exploitation.**

Name: ____________________ Surname: ____________________

Country: ____________________ Date: ____________________

E-mail address: ____________________

**Q1 Is elder maltreatment a problem in your country?**

- ☐ It is a very big problem
- ☐ It is a big problem
- ☐ It is a moderate problem
- ☐ It is a slight problem
- ☐ It is not a problem at all

**Q2 Is elder maltreatment perceived as a problem in your country?**

- ☐ It is perceived as a very big problem
- ☐ It is perceived as a big problem
- ☐ It is perceived as a moderate problem
- ☐ It is perceived as a slight problem
- ☐ It is not perceived as a problem at all

**Q3 Is there a national policy in your country on elder maltreatment?**

☐ YES ☐ YES, in some areas ☐ NO

**Q3.1 If yes, can you provide a hard/electronic copy/a web link?**

**Q4 Have the following evidence-based interventions implemented in your country?**

**Q4.1 Encouraging positive attitudes toward older people through the use of education programmes for health care workers**

☐ YES ☐ YES, in some areas ☐ NO

**Q4.2 Increasing support for informal caregivers through the use of peer and professional support groups (To allow carers to discuss problems with people in similar situations, increase their social network and gain information and advice about caregiving and caring responsibilities)**

☐ YES ☐ YES, in some areas ☐ NO

**Q4.3 Respite programmes (they provide care for an elderly dependent person to give caregivers a break from the burden of their responsibilities)**

☐ YES ☐ YES, in some areas ☐ NO

**Q4.4** **Psychological programmes offered to carers to lessen emotional distress (These can include anger and depression management, cognitive behavioural therapy and can be offered to those experiencing psychological problems or those who have abused or neglected their elderly dependents)**

☐ YES ☐ YES, in some areas ☐ NO

**Q4.5** **Increasing identification and referral for victims of maltreatment (through the use of screening tools and training for health and other professionals)**

☐ YES ☐ YES, in some areas ☐ NO

**Q4.6** **Supporting victims of maltreatment (through multi-agency work to ensure efficient reporting and management of elder maltreatment cases in the community)**

☐ YES ☐ YES, in some areas ☐ NO

**Q4.7** **Is there any other kind of intervention implemented?**

☐ YES ☐ NO ☐ I don't know

**Q4.7.1 If YES, please specify**

**Q5** **Is data on elder maltreatment collected in your country?**

☐ YES ☐ NO ☐ I don't know

**Q5.1** **If you answer yes to Q5, can you please specify? (a multiple answer is allowed)**

☐ Community survey

☐ Health facility data

☐ Residential facility data

☐ Other, please specify below

**Q5.2** **If you answer yes to Q5, how was elder maltreatment defined?**

**Q5.3** **If you answer yes to Q5, can you please provide a hard/electronic copy/a web link of document(s) reporting this?**

**Q5.4** **If it is not in English, please try to provide a short summary in a separate file**

**Q6** **Are there studies in your country estimating the proportion of homicides in the elderly due to elder maltreatment?**

☐ YES ☐ NO ☐ I don't know

**Q7** **Are you interested in having more information on elder maltreatment?**

☐ YES ☐ NO

**Q8** **Is there any research institute/university in your country concerned with elder maltreatment?**

☐ YES ☐ NO

**Q9** **If yes, can you please provide their details**

**Thank you for your collaboration!**

# Annex 4. Health ministry focal people for violence prevention and other respondents to the survey

| | |
|---|---|
| Albania | Gentiana Qirjako, Public Health Department |
| Andorra | Rosa Vidal, Ministry of Health, Labour and Welfare |
| Armenia | Ruzanna Yuzbashyan, Ministry of Health |
| Austria | Maria Orthofer, Federal Ministry of Economy, Family and Youth |
| Azerbaijan | Rustam Talishinskiy, Traumatology Centre Baku |
| Belgium | Christiane Hauzeur, Federal Public Service for Health, Food Chain Safety and Environment |
| Bosnia and Herzegovina[a] | Alen Seranic, Ministry of Health and Social Welfare, Republic of Srpska |
| Bulgaria | Fanka Koycheva, National Center for Public Health Protection |
| Croatia | Ivana Bkrić Biloš, Croatian National Institute of Public Health |
| Cyprus | Myrto Azina-Chronidou, Ministry of Health |
| Czech Republic | Iva Truellova, Ministry of Health |
| Denmark | Karin Helweg-Larsen, National Institute of Public Health |
| Estonia | Kristiina Luht and Külli Pärnpuu-Kasemaa, Ministry of Social Affairs |
| Finland | Heidi Manns-Haatanen, Ministry of Social Affairs and Health |
| Germany | Robert Schüßler, Federal Ministry of Health |
| Greece | Anastasia Ntina Zygoura, Hellenic National Center for Emergency Care |
| Hungary | Maria Herczog, Eszterházy Károly College |
| Iceland | Rosa Thorsteinsdottir, Public Health Institute of Iceland |
| Ireland | Robbie Breen, Health Promotion Policy Unit, Department of Health and Children |

[a] Only the Republic of Srpska.

| | |
|---|---|
| Israel | Kobi Peleg, Israel National Center for Trauma and Emergency Medicine; Barbara Lang, Aaron Cohen and Iris Rasooly, Ministry of Health |
| Italy | Maria Giuseppina Lecce, Ministry of Health |
| Latvia | Jana Feldmane, Ministry of Health |
| Lithuania | Robertas Povilaitis, Childline |
| Malta | Taygeta Firman, General Directorate for Health |
| Montenegro | Svetlana Stojanovic, Ministry of Health |
| Netherlands | Loek J.W. Hesemans, Ministry of Health, Welfare and Sport |
| Norway | Freja Ulvestad Kärki, Norwegian Directorate of Health |
| Portugal | Maria João Quintela, Directorate-General of Health |
| Romania | Daniel Verman, Ministry of Health |
| Russian Federation | Margarita Kachaeva, Centre for Social and Forensic Psychiatry |
| San Marino | Andrea Gualtieri, Authority of Public Health |
| Serbia | Milena Paunovic, Institute of Public Health of Belgrade |
| Slovakia | Martin Smrek, University Children's Hospital; Barbara Holubova, Kvetoslava Repkova, Institute of Labour and Family Research; Beata Balogova, University of Presov |
| Slovenia | Barbara Mihevc Ponikvar, Institute for Public Health |
| Spain | Begoña Merino, Ministry of Health and Social Policy |
| Switzerland | Marie-Claude Hofner, University Institute for Legal Medicine |
| Tajikistan | Gulbakhor Ashurova and Saodat Kamalova, Ministry of Health |
| The former Yugoslav Republic of Macedonia | Marija Raleva, Clinic for Psychiatry, Clinical Center Skopje |
| United Kingdom | Mark Bellis and Sarah Wood, Liverpool John Moores University |
| Uzbekistan | Alisher Iskandarov, Pediatric Medical Institute |